SECRET OF HEALTHY HAIR

Your Complete Food & Lifestyle Guide for Healthy Hair with Season Wise Diet Plans and Hair Care Recipes

LA FONCEUR

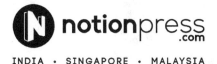

INDIA · SINGAPORE · MALAYSIA

Notion Press

Old No. 38, New No. 6
McNichols Road, Chetpet
Chennai - 600 031

First Published by Notion Press 2019
Copyright © La Fonceur 2019
All Rights Reserved.

ISBN 978-1-64650-671-2

This book has been published with all efforts taken to make the material error-free after the consent of the author. However, the author and the publisher do not assume and hereby disclaim any liability to any party for any loss, damage, or disruption caused by errors or omissions, whether such errors or omissions result from negligence, accident, or any other cause.

While every effort has been made to avoid any mistake or omission, this publication is being sold on the condition and understanding that neither the author nor the publishers or printers would be liable in any manner to any person by reason of any mistake or omission in this publication or for any action taken or omitted to be taken or advice rendered or accepted on the basis of this work. For any defect in printing or binding the publishers will be liable only to replace the defective copy by another copy of this work then available.

La Fouceur

CONTENTS

Preface   7

Introduction   9

1. Everything about Hair   11

1. Everything about Hair – Hair Structure, Hair Color, and Hair Growth   13

    Hair Structure   15

    Reason for Different Hair Color   17

    Hair Growth Cycle   19

2. 10 Most Important Nutrients for Hair Health   21
3. 10 Worst Foods You Should Avoid for Healthy Hair   30
4. 10 Everyday Bad Habits That Are Damaging Your Hair   38
5. 10 Healthy Habits for Smoother, Shinier, Stronger, and Healthier Hair   47
6. Top 10 Foods for Smoother, Shinier, Stronger, and Healthier Hair   57
7. Top 10 Foods that Prevent Hair Loss and Promote Hair Growth   69

2. Hair Problems, Their Reasons, and Their Solutions   79

1. Hair Problems, Their Reasons, and Their Solutions Part 1   81

    Gray/White Hair   82

    Dandruff   83

    Split Ends   85

Frizzy Hair	87
Tangled Hair	90
2. Hair Problems, Their Reasons, and Their Solutions Part 2	93
Hair Fall	94
Head Lice	97
Greasy Hair	99
Dry Hair	101
3. Diet Plan & Lifestyle Guide Season Wise	**105**
Winter	107
Lifestyle Guide	107
Diet Plan	108
Summer	109
Lifestyle Guide	109
Diet Plan	110
Monsoon	111
Lifestyle Guide	111
Diet Plan	112
4. Recipes	**113**
Bean Salad	115
Crunchy Chocolate Oats Drops	117
Palak Paneer	120
Sesame, Peanut, and Coconut Chikki	124
About the Author	127
Note from La Fonceur	128
Other Books by La Fonceur	129
Connect with La Fonceur	130

PREFACE

Hair loss, bad hair, split ends, and many more hair related problems! I was receiving lots of emails from my blog readers to write about the vegetarian foods that can be included in the diet to combat hair problems. Bad hair equals a bad day. Whether man or woman, no one is unfamiliar to this, including me. Being a health-conscious person as well as a researcher by profession, even a sneeze makes me think, what's the underlying reason of it? I believe in solving the problem by working on the root cause because when you work on the root cause, you can influence the final result.

Being from the pharma field, everyone asks me about medication for hair loss or other hair problems. But I would suggest, medicines should be your last option for your hair problems, until and unless you have massive hair fall or other severe hair issues because these signs could be due to other internal health problems.

Food therapy is the best therapy. In this book, I am going to discuss, with the right food choices and some healthy habits how most of your hair problems can be solved. When you eat right hair nutrients and follow some secret hair routines, you get shinier, smoother, stronger, and healthier hair. I have also included some recipes in this book; the best part is, each and every ingredient of these recipes contributes to your hair growth. In fact, some of them are my original recipes, I make them quite frequently, and they are part of my regular diet.

If you have tried everything for your hair from taking various hair treatments to applying every hair mask trending on the internet and still wondering why your hair is still NOT healthy? Then **Secret of Healthy Hair** book is for you!

La Fonceur
30/July/2019

INTRODUCTION

Hair related problems are something that everyone experience in his/her life at some point. This could be related to hair loss, premature graying, or overall hair quality. Our hair can be damaged due to many reasons. Our daily routine affects our hair health. What we eat, how we feel, how well we take care of our hair, these all factors hugely affect our hair health as well as its growth. Different people have different hair problems, but what are the exact causes of these problems? Why do some people have dry hair while others have split end problems? Why can't some people grow their hair after a certain length? What are the underlying causes of that? How can you influence your hair health and its growth rate? How can you get rid of these problems permanently? How can you get smoother, shiner, and stronger hair that you always dreamt about?

These all questions will be answered in this book. When you exactly know what are you doing wrong, you can work on it. Working on the root cause instead of superficially hiding your hair flaws will give you a permanent lifelong solution to your hair problems.

This book will explain how by including right hair nutrients in your diet and following some simple hair care routines, you can get control over your hair problems and have the world's healthiest and strongest hair. This book also includes the customized lifestyle and diet plan for winter, summer, and monsoon season. You will also find some healthy and yummy recipes in which each and every ingredient contributes to hair health.

This book is your complete hair guide which you can carry with you everywhere you go. Whenever in doubt, open this hair guide, check out what you need to do for your hair problem and you are ready to rock the world.

1
EVERYTHING ABOUT HAIR

1
EVERYTHING ABOUT HAIR – HAIR STRUCTURE, HAIR COLOR, AND HAIR GROWTH

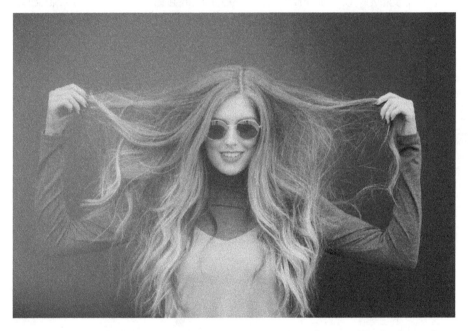

Everything About Hair – Hair Structure, Hair Color, and Hair Growth

What does your hair mean to you? Probably your most powerful and beautiful asset! Hair and beauty have a deep relationship. Hair is one of the defining characteristics of women and men. A bad hair day means a bad day. For some, their hair is a form of personal expression. You must have noticed that you feel super confident the day you have beautiful hair. You naturally feel that I can conquer the world, all because my hair is shiny, smoothly flowing, and looks amazing today! Healthy hair gives a confidence boost while bad hair really ruins the mood and enthusiasm.

In this book, I am going to discuss all things about hair, what foods and factors positively or negatively affect your hair, and what are the solutions. But first, let's see what hair is actually made of and how it works?

HAIR STRUCTURE

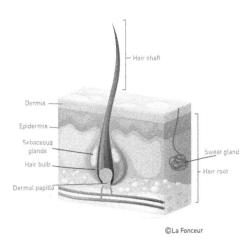

Hair is made up of keratin, a tough protein.

Hair Follicle

Hair grows from follicles found in the dermis layer of skin; these follicles are called hair follicles, in simple terms, the part of hair beneath the skin called as the hair follicle.

Hair Shaft

The part of the hair that can be seen above your scalp is called hair shaft. The hair shaft is comprised of three layers: cuticle, cortex, and medulla.

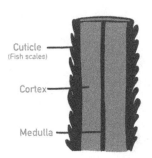

Cuticle: The cuticle is the outer most protective layer of the hair which has a fish scale (facing downwards) likes cells that overlap. These cells prevent damage to the cortex, hair's inner structure. It also controls the moisture content of hair fiber.

Cuticle gives your hair shine and protects the inner layers from the damage. However, excessive heat, chemical over-processing, and weather change can damage the protective cuticle layer of the hair, affecting the integrity of the hair.

Cortex: The middle layer called cortex is the main component of the hair. It consists of long keratin chains that add bulk, strength, and elasticity to the hair. The health of your cortex depends mainly on how well the cuticle is protecting it.

Cortex also contains the pigment melanin. Melanin is the pigment responsible for giving hair its natural color. Hair coloring, relaxing, thermal styling, and other aggressive treatments cause temporary or permanent changes to the cortex layer.

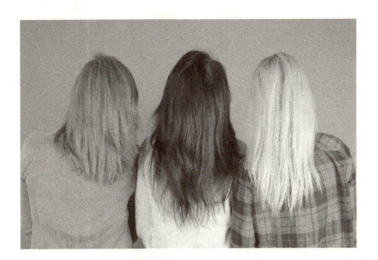

REASON FOR DIFFERENT HAIR COLOR

There are two types of melanin found in the hair cortex layer:

Eumelanin is responsible for black and brown hair color.

Pheomelanin is responsible for blonde, red, and yellow hair color.

Gray or white hair happens because of an absence of melanin pigment in the cortex layer, which can be due to age or other factors.

Medulla: The innermost layer of the hair shaft, the medulla is composed of an amorphous, and round cell. This layer is generally absent, especially within naturally blonde and fine hair and normally present in thicker, coarser and darker hair.

This was all about hair shaft, the part of the hair that can be seen above your scalp. Now let's see what happens beneath the skin.

Intense biochemical and metabolic activity that develops beneath the epidermis is responsible for development and hair growth.

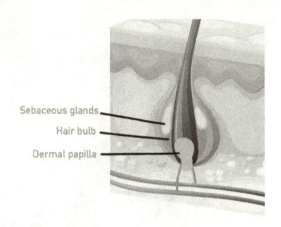

Hair Bulb

The hair bulb contains stem cells that divide and grow new hair follicles that build the hair shaft. The cone-shaped dermal papilla in the hair bulb contains the blood supply and nerves that nourish the cells and deliver nutrients to the hair.

Sebaceous Glands

Sebaceous glands or oil glands attached to hair follicles release an oily or waxy secretion called sebum that lubricates and waterproof the hair. Sebum gives a natural shine to your hair and protects it from bacteria. Thick hair contains more number of sebaceous glands.

HAIR GROWTH CYCLE

Hair growth rates are different in different people; it depends on age, hair type, and hair health. Hair grows at an average of around one-half inch (1.25 cm) per month; this means about 6 inches of hair per year. Every hair can be at a different stage of the growth cycle at any given time.

Let's see what are these phases and how long do they last.

Anagen (growth phase)

Duration: 2–3 years (Maximum 7 years)

Anagen is the active growing phase of hair follicles during which cell in the root of the hair is dividing rapidly, forming a new hair. Normally 90–95% of the hair follicles are in the anagen phase. Hair stays in this growth phase for two to a maximum of seven years.

Catagen (transition or regressing phase)

2–3 weeks (Approx. 10 days)

Catagen is a short transition stage. It signals the end of the anagen phase during which growth stops and the hair follicle shrinks, the outer root sheath attaches to the root of the hair and detaches from the dermal papilla. This forms a bulge at the end, that is known as a club hair. Catagen phase lasts for about 2–3 weeks and about 1–2% of all hairs are in the catagen phase.

Telogen (resting phase)

2–3 months (Around 100 days)

The telogen phase is the resting phase during which hair follicle is completely at rest, and the final product of a hair follicle, the club hair is completely formed. A club hair is a dead, fully keratinized hair, and if you pull out a hair in the telogen phase, it will reveal a solid, dry, white bulge at the root. This phase lasts for about 100 days, and about 10–14% of the hair are in the telogen phase at any time.

Exogen (shedding phase)

This phase is characterized by the departure of a club hair from the scalp that results in hair shedding. Exogen phase accounts for the 100–150 hairs fall out every day. Anything that disrupts the hair growth cycle, such as hair relaxing, coloring, excessive heat can cause more hairs to enter the telogen phase then in a few months hair enters the exogen phase, and a greater amount of hair shed.

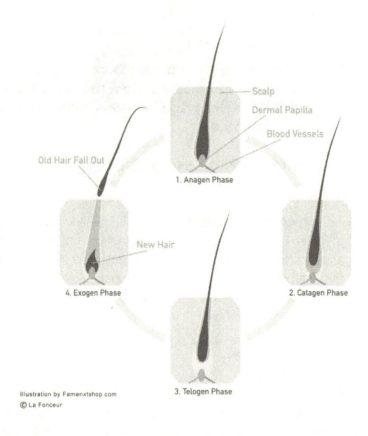

Hair Growth Cycle

2
10 MOST IMPORTANT NUTRIENTS FOR HAIR HEALTH

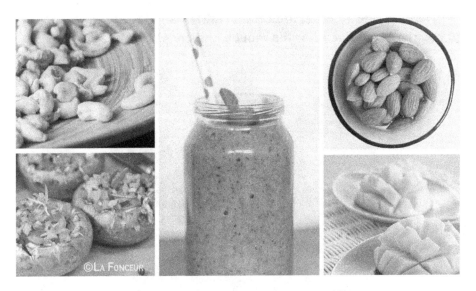

10 Most Important Nutrients for Hair Health

Yes, a healthy diet can be the solution to most of the hair problems, even including hair loss. Diet low in nutrients, may cause dry, brittle, and rough hair. Coarse and brittle hair could be a sign of iron deficiency anemia. Vitamin B12 deficiency can cause premature graying. A lack of protein in your diet promote hair loss.

With the right nutrients in your diet, you can hugely influence your hair quality. A healthy diet is a key to silky, shiny, radiant, and fuller hair.

Here are the 10 Most Important Nutrients for Your Hair to include in your diet that can offer the most significant benefits:

1. Protein

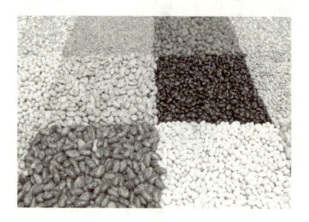

Eating enough protein is essential for healthy and strong hair. Protein promotes hair growth because hair follicles are made of mostly protein called keratin. The protein-rich diet helps the body to produce keratin, which is fundamental to the hair structure. When keratin weakens, hair strands become dry and brittle. One should eat high protein and iron-rich diet to prevent hair loss.

Read 10 High Protein Sources For Vegetarians and 10 Reasons You Should Eat More Protein Every Day in the previous book **Eat So What! The Power of Vegetarianism (Full Version).**

2. Iron

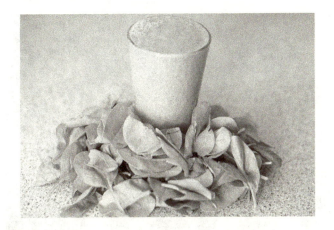

Iron deficiency can cause anemia, which is a major cause of hair loss in men or women. Without enough iron, the body can't produce enough hemoglobin in red blood cells. Hemoglobin is the main part of red blood cells and binds oxygen. Hemoglobin in the blood carries oxygen from the lungs or gills for the repair and growth of cells in the body, including the cells responsible for stimulating and maintaining the hair growth.

Simultaneous consumption of vitamin C increases the absorption of non-heme iron. Try to combine non-heme iron foods with vitamin C (for example, a glass of lemon juice, oranges, and berries) to increase absorption of iron.

Read 10 Power Foods To Get Rid Of Anemia in the previous book **Eat So What! The Power of Vegetarianism Volume 2 (Mini Edition).**

3. Vitamin B12

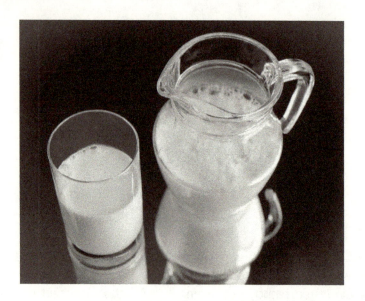

Vitamin B12, or cobalamin, is one of the essential water-soluble vitamins. Deficiency in vitamin B12 can contribute to premature graying. Vitamin B12 is a cofactor in DNA synthesis. Body needs vitamin B12 for fatty acid and amino acid metabolism. It assists in red blood cell production and responsible for producing new hair cells. Deficiency in vitamin B12 can lead to anemia that impacts hair growth process and is one of the common reason for hair fall. Premature graying or hair fall due to vitamin B12 deficiency is reversible if you increase your intake of vitamin B12.

Read Top 10 Foods For Vegetarians To Prevent Vitamin B12 Deficiency in the previous book **Eat So What! The Power of Vegetarianism Volume 1 (Mini Edition)**.

4. Vitamin D

Research shows that people with hair loss have much lower vitamin D levels than people who do not have hair loss problem. Vitamin D deficiency can cause hair loss and other hair problems. Vitamin D stimulates new and old hair follicles to grow.

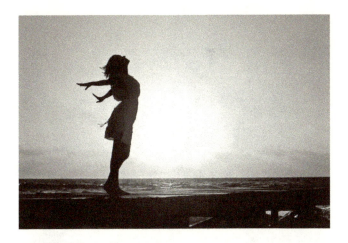

When body does not have enough vitamin D, hair growth may be stunted. Vitamin D can be synthesized by the body when the skin gets exposed to ultraviolet rays from sunlight. Take 10–25 minutes of early morning sun exposure every day.

5. Omega-3 Fats

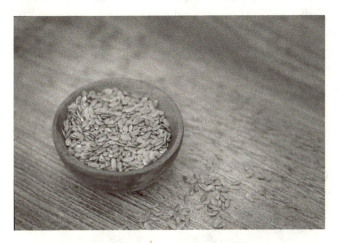

Omega-3 fats reduce inflammation, dry flaky scalp, nourish hair, and promote healthy hair. Lack of omega-3 fatty acids in the body can lead to dry, opaque, and brittle hair, which can cause dandruff. Omega-3 fats moisturize hair follicles that add elasticity, shine, and brightness to your hair. Diet rich in omega-3 and omega-6 fatty acids reduce hair loss and increase hair density.

6. Zinc

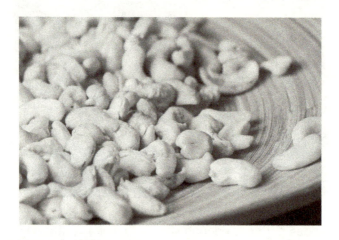

Zinc plays a vital role in tissue repair and hair growth. Alopecia is a sign of zinc deficiency. Zinc inhibits the transformation of testosterone into DHT (dihydrotestosterone) hormone that causes alopecia. Zinc is also essential to produce sebum, which is the natural oil secreted by the scalp that helps in keeping the hair silky and strengthening the hair follicles. Zinc deficiency may lead to dull hair and even lead to hair loss. Always soak beans and pulses overnight because cereal grains contain phytic acid that reduces zinc absorption. Soaking these foods reduce phytic acids present in them.

7. Biotin

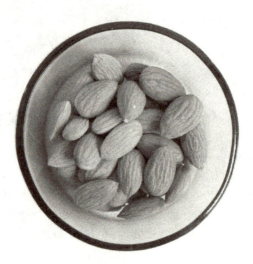

Biotin is a water-soluble vitamin B7 and also known as vitamin H or coenzyme R. Hair loss and hair thinning are the symptoms of biotin deficiency. Biotin is a coenzyme that enhances enzymes activity involved in metabolizing carbohydrates and fats, influencing tissue growth, including hair tissues. Biotin affects amino acids involved in protein synthesis, supporting your hair health. Biotin influence hair growth and give thickness and strength to your hair.

8. Selenium

Selenium is an essential trace element that means the body cannot synthesize it, and you have to take in through dietary source. Selenium plays a vital role in the synthesis of more than 35 proteins. Selenium deficiency is involved in hair graying during childhood or early adulthood. Eating selenium-rich foods improve premature graying, dandruff, and dry scalp and promote healthy hair growth.

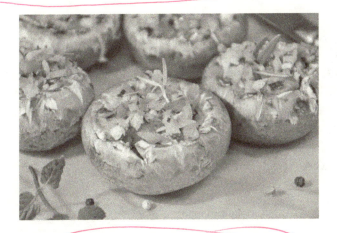

Selenium sources: Beans, mushroom, nuts, and seeds.

9. Vitamin E

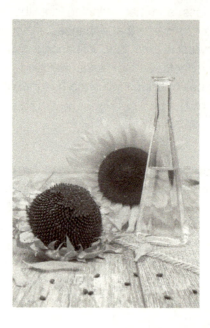

Vitamin E is responsible for maintaining scalp health. It has natural antioxidant effects that fight free radicals. It reduces inflammation that causes the hair follicle cells to break down, hence, prevent hair loss, and maintain hair health. Vitamin E locks moisture, gives you shiny, strong, healthy hair and protects your hair from drying out.

10. Vitamin A

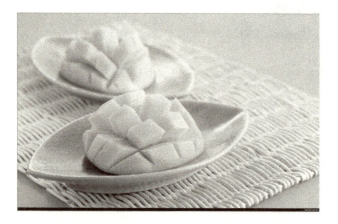

Vitamin A is essential for healthy hair. Vitamin A is essential for growth and cells repairment, including hair cells. Vitamin A also helps skin glands produce sebum, the natural oil which is responsible for keeping the scalp moisturized and hair healthy. This fat-soluble vitamin nourishes hair, stimulates hair growth, and prevents the dry, brittle hair. However, too much of vitamin A can also contribute to hair loss.

CONCLUSION

Poor diet affects overall hair health. Diet lack in important hair nutrients can cause breaking and thin hair. Premature graying and hair loss can be the indication of anemia, vitamin B12, and vitamin D deficiencies, low selenium, and zinc levels. Hair loss due to nutrient deficiency is reversible if you increase your intake of the deficient vitamins and minerals.

3
10 WORST FOODS YOU SHOULD AVOID FOR HEALTHY HAIR

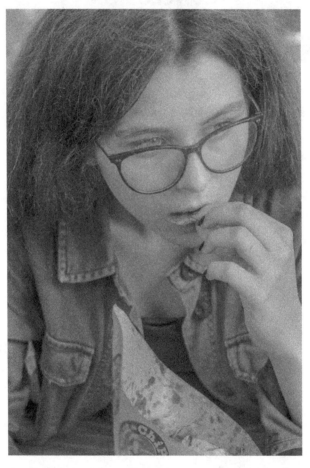

10 Worst Foods You Should Avoid for Healthy Hair

It takes more than good shampoo and conditioner to help your hair look its best. Your hair gets affected by the foods you eat. Your hair tells how well or poorly you are feeding your body. Poor diet may cause loss of hair or make your hair dull, brittle, and thin. Of course, several other lifestyle choices also play an essential role in affecting your hair health, including smoking, and how often do you oil your hair but by eating nutrient-rich foods and avoiding those that only harm, you can influence your hair growth, volume, shine and its likelihood of graying.

Below are 10 Worst Foods for Hair You Should Avoid:

1. Sugar

Sugar is not good for your hair; it promotes inflammation. High sugar intake spikes blood sugar levels, causing a spike of insulin and androgens, which then bind to hair follicles and potentially accelerate hair loss. It doesn't mean you need to stop having sugar completely; it is generally seen in people who chronically have high levels of insulin. Over the long term, when high sugar intakes consistently drive inflammation, it affects the immune system and overall affects hair health.

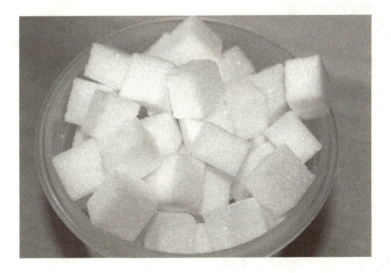

If you are a sweet tooth, try adding some fresh fruits in your diet as they satiate your sweet craving as well as nourish your body.

2. Alcohol

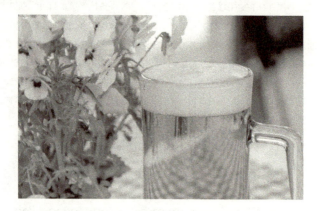

Any alcoholic beverages, including spirits, beer, and wine, interfere with metabolization of zinc and cause a reduction of the zinc level in the body. Zinc is a crucial mineral that plays a vital role in your hair growth. When zinc level is too low, it stops hair growth, and hair fall may start. Alcohol also dehydrates you and can make your hair brittle, dry, and more prone to breakage.

3. Starchy Food

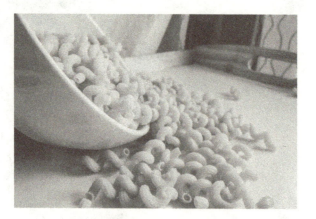

Foods such as cake, white bread, and pasta, contain starch. Processed starches are quickly broken down into sugar in the body and cause thinning of hair. Research has also shown that starchy food can increase androgen levels, particularly an androgen called dihydrotestosterone (DHT) that can lead to a shorter cycle of hair growth and cause hair follicles to become thinner. So, have such foods only in moderation and stick with whole wheat whenever possible.

4. Salt

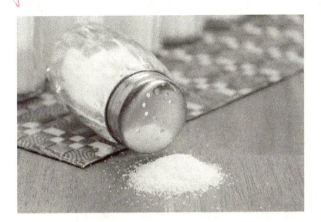

Salt should be consumed moderately. Side effects of taking an excessive amount of salt are not only limited to kidney problems, and high blood pressure, but it can wreak havoc on your hair too. Salt is considered as harmful for hair as it contains sodium which has its own side effects. So, always opt for low sodium and low salt diet. You should go for sea salt which is another form of salt that contains 26 minerals which give your hair a better shine, volume, and strength as it intensifies blood circulation in the scalp that boosts hair growth.

5. Diet Soda

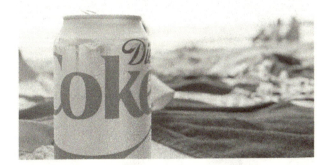

Diet soda contains artificial sweetener, like aspartame, which is not good for your hair. Aspartame can cause hair loss and hair fall. Not only bad for hair, but aspartame can also cause depression, arthritis, impotency, and bloating. Staying completely away from such drinks will keep your hair shiny and healthy. You can switch from diet soda to natural healthy drinks to stay hydrated.

6. Lack of Zinc and Iron

Zinc plays a vital role in hair growth and repair. Zinc inhibits the DHT hormone that causes alopecia. Zinc is also essential to produce sebum, which is the natural oil secreted by the scalp that helps in keeping the hair healthy and strengthening the hair follicles. Zinc deficiency may lead to dull hair and even lead to hair loss.

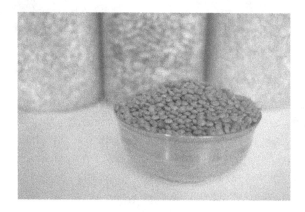

Lack of iron means your body can't produce enough hemoglobin in your blood. This red protein is responsible for transporting oxygen in the blood for growth and repair of cells, including the cells that stimulate hair growth. Iron deficiency may lead to hair loss.

7. Insufficient Protein

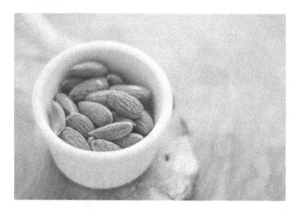

Eating enough protein is important for healthy and strong hair. Protein promotes hair growth because hair follicles are made of the protein keratin. Keratin helps to keep your hair healthy. Protein-rich diet helps the body to produce keratin, which is fundamental to the hair structure. When keratin weakens, hair strands become dry and brittle.

8. Greasy Food

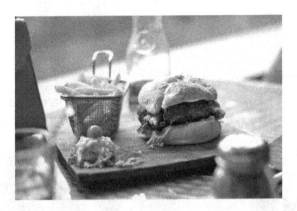

Foods that are high in saturated fats and trans fats not only can clog the arteries, even clog the sweat pores on your scalp and also cause greasy hair. As the pores of the scalp get clogged, the harmful hormones get trapped, which can trigger the hair loss mechanism. Avoid foods which are high in saturated fat such as hard margarine, butter, and fried foods.

9. Too Much of Vitamin A

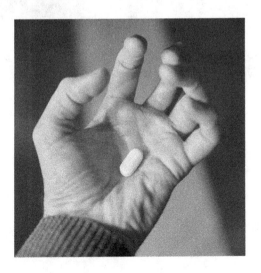

While Vitamin A helps skin glands to produce sebum, the natural oily substance that moisturizes the scalp and helps keep hair healthy. Overloading with vitamin A can cause hair loss and can be toxic to the hair follicles. Excessive Vitamin A in the body can shrink the oil gland; as a result, oil gland may not produce the same amount of oil which is necessary to coat the hair and make it shiny and healthy.

That doesn't mean you should stop eating carrots as it takes millions of carrots to result in excessive vitamin A in the body, it is generally seen in the people who take lots of vitamin supplements that can damage the hair.

10. Carbonated Drinks

Carbonated drinks are quite acid forming. They are also loaded with excessive sugar, which spikes blood sugar levels and then crashes.

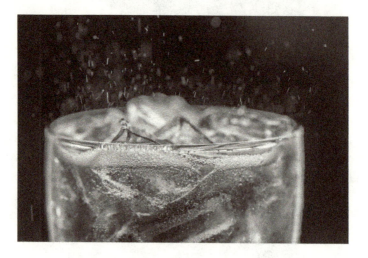

Many studies show the link between excess blood sugar and male pattern baldness. It is advisable to avoid carbonated drinks as much as you can.

CONCLUSION

Who doesn't want shiny, strong, and healthy hair? Your hair needs complete nutrition. Unhealthy diets can result in dry, brittle, lackluster hair. When the body doesn't get enough nutrition such as protein, biotin, zinc, iron, and other nutrients that it needs from the diet, it can result in loss of hair. If you are experiencing hair loss, then pay attention to your diet, what you ate in about two to three months. Is your diet protein-deficient or lack of iron, zinc? Or maybe your diet is full of unhealthy foods that are nutritionless and damaging your hair health. Putting restriction to these unhealthy foods for some months as well as adding more nutritious food in your diet may help you get your lustrous waves back.

4
10 EVERYDAY BAD HABITS THAT ARE DAMAGING YOUR HAIR

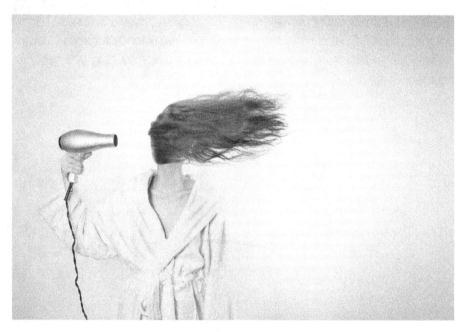

10 Everyday Bad Habits That Are Damaging Your Hair

Sometimes we do things unintentionally in our daily routine that are actually hurting our hair health. The health of your hair depends on how well you take care of yourself. Many aspects of lifestyle, from the food you eat to the way you style your hair can impact the quality of your hair. While certain health problems, medication, stress, and genetics have a direct connection to our hair health, there might be many everyday bad habits that can wreak havoc on your hair.

Here are 10 Everyday Bad Habits That Are Hurting Your Hair Health:

1. Detangling Wet Hair

When your hair is wet, it swells and loses its strength, which causes hair to break off even under the low pressure. So, your wet strands are far more fragile than dry hair. Brushing wet hair with a fine-tooth comb can all lead to breakage.

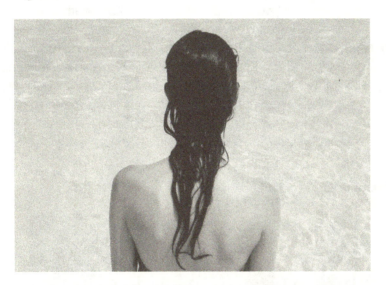

For extra protection, apply conditioner after shampoo to reduce friction between strands of hair that allow easier brushing. It's better to let your hair dry naturally and comb when it's dry.

2. Taking Hot Showers

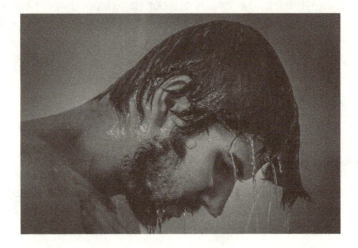

We all enjoy hot showers, especially when the weather is cool. No doubt, hot shower instantly makes us feel great and relaxed, but at the same time, it is not good for your hair. Avoid washing your hair with excessively hot water. Rinsing with hot water results in temporary inflammation of the scalp and you may experience pain and skin redness as well as it takes away natural oils from your scalp leaving your scalp dehydrated. Always rinse with cold water after a hot shower; otherwise, your weaker strands may start breaking off.

3. Overexposure to Sun

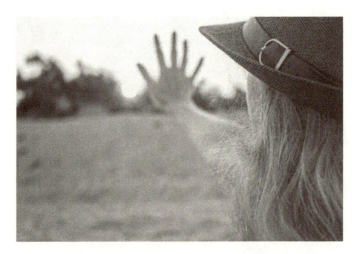

Just like your skin, your hair also needs protection from harsh UVA and UVB rays. If you expose your hair to the sun for long periods of time, UVA and UVB rays can damage the hair cuticle (the outermost part of the hair shaft) and dehydrate your locks. Signs of sun damage include changes in the color, look, and texture of your hair. Damaged hair has a dry look, split ends, frizziness, thinning and brittle strands. Use shampoo which gives UV protection. Get your hair trimmed to get rid of split ends.

4. Tying Up Your Hair Tightly

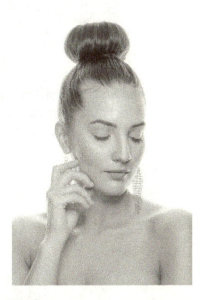

When you tie up your hair too tightly, then the elastic exerts too much pressure, and the constant pulling can cause strands of your hair to break or even fall out, which, in the long, can damage your hair follicles. This can result in Traction Alopecia, which is a form of alopecia, or gradual hair loss, caused primarily by pulling pressure being applied to the hair. To avoid damage, pick hair ties that are covered with fabric and use bobby pins or hair clips when you need to get your hair out of your face.

5. Using Same Hair Products After Hair Treatment

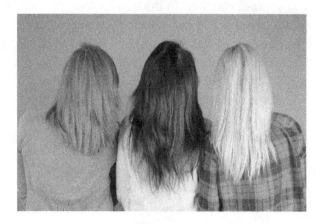

If you have done hair treatment, whether highlights or keratin treatment, don't use your regular shampoo or conditioner. Your regular shampoo contains harsh chemicals like sodium lauryl sulfate (SLS) that depletes natural oils and hair proteins and sodium chloride (salt) which are abrasive in nature. Your treated hair will look healthier and last longer with the proper shampoo and conditioner.

6. Washing Your Hair Too Frequently

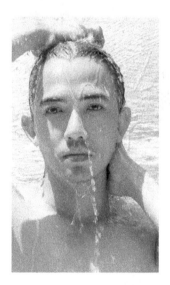

Washing your hair every day does not cause hair loss but removes sebum, which is the natural oil secreted by sebaceous glands. Sebum keeps the hair moisturized and stripping it can lead to dull, dry, and brittle locks. Moisturized hair looks healthy and shiny and is less likely to break or look frizzy and dry. If you have dry hair type, you should shampoo a maximum of two times a week.

7. Vigorously Towel Drying Your Wet Hair

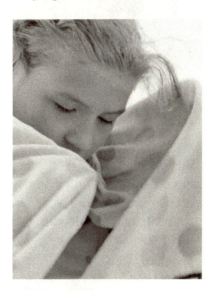

Wet hair is weak and more prone to breakage. Vigorously rubbing your wet hair with a cotton or terry cloth towel can cause friction, which can lead to excessive hair breakage, frizz, and hair fall. Air drying is the healthiest way to let your wet hair dry. Instead of vigorously rubbing, blot and squeeze your hair with a microfiber towel. Microfiber towels are super absorbent and don't need much rubbing.

8. Overheating Your Hair

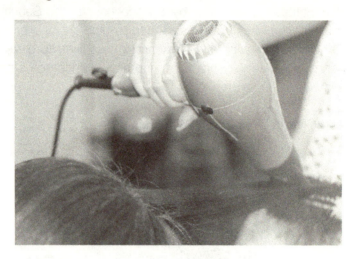

Though wet hair is more prone to breakage that doesn't mean you have to blow dry your hair every time. Let your hair air dry naturally; do not blow dry your hair too often. Using a blow dryer on high or using hot straighteners or curling irons every day dehydrates your hair, leaving it dull and prone to damage. The high temperatures of these devices weaken the fibers of your hair. Avoid overheating your hair and use a spray-in heat protectant when using such devices.

9. Over Exposer to Chemicals

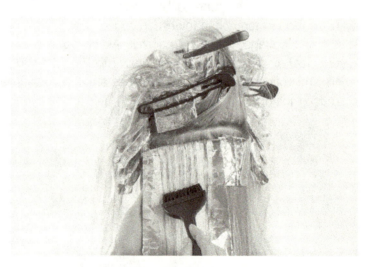

Do not dye, perm, or bleach your hair frequently. Constant perming, coloring, bleaching, and relaxing expose your hair to a lot of chemicals. Permanent hair colors contain harsh chemicals, such as ammonia, which can lead to drier and weaker hair. Hair may break if you overdo on chemical processes, this may also cause scalp burns. Increase the time between hair treatments, such as perms and dyes. Always remember to inform your hairdresser in advance about any previous treatments so that they can pick the best and safe treatments for your hair.

10. Continuous Touching Your Hair

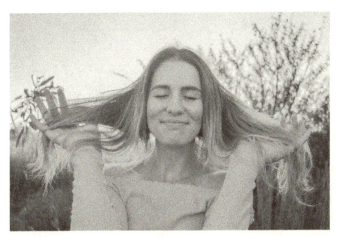

Playing with your hair may be a way of flirting but overdoing it may harm your hair health. If you have the bad habit of regularly touching your hair throughout the day, then you need to control it. Your hands touch a lot of things throughout the day; they accumulate dirt and oils. If you play with your hair, then the dirt and oils of your fingers can mix in with the natural oils in your hair, not only that, they can actually steal away natural oils that make your hair look good, leading to dry, frizzy and easily broken hair strands.

CONCLUSION

With some precautions such as using a shampoo with UV protectant, avoiding excessive hot water shower, avoiding overheating your hair, and increasing the time between hair treatments or just by minutely changing the way you handle your hair like using microfiber towel instead of cotton towel, combing the hair when it's dry, you can get stronger, shinier and healthier hair. So, say goodbye to the bad hair habits, and you will never have a bad hair day again.

5
10 HEALTHY HABITS FOR SMOOTHER, SHINIER, STRONGER, AND HEALTHIER HAIR

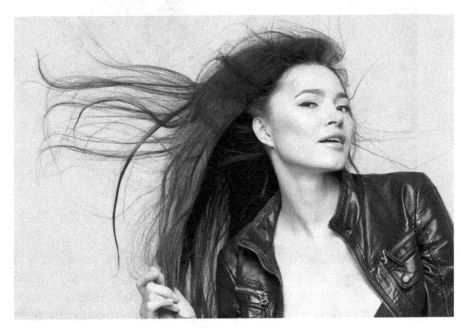

10 Healthy Habits for Smoother, Shinier, Stronger, and Healthier Hair

Different factors affect how silky, strong, and healthy your hair is. It all depends on how well you take care of your hair. We all want strong and healthy hair, but it needs proper care and nourishment. Just by following simple healthy habits you can have the hair you have always dreamt about.

From eating right nutrients rich diet, to regularly oiling your hair, here are the some of the simple healthy habits you can use to encourage hair growth and get smoother, stronger, shinier and healthier hair.

1. Trim Your Hair Every Two to Three Months

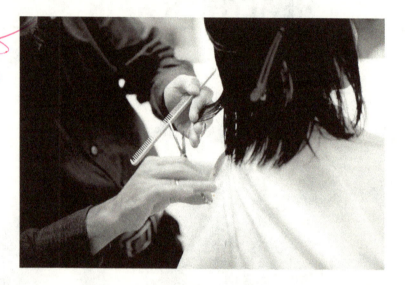

Haircuts help to maintain hair health. Although it seems the last thing, you would consider when you are trying to grow out your hair. However, trimming your hair every two to three months while growing it out, actually encourage hair growth by getting rid of split ends, breakage, and damaged hair. Trimming ensures minimal split ends or breakage and results in fuller and healthier hair.

2. Comb Every Day

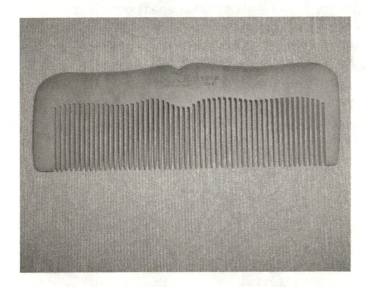

Combing every day is good for your hair. Massage your scalp every day with a wooden-bristle brush to stimulate the hair growth. Pressure applied by wooden-bristle brush activates blood circulation to the hair follicles, and that channels more nutrients to the hair roots, conditions the scalp and stimulates hair growth.

3. Use Sulfate-Free Shampoo

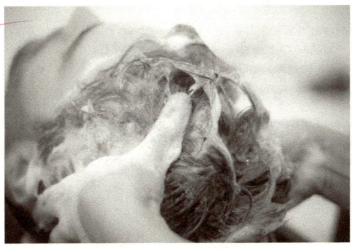

Sodium lauryl sulfate and Sodium dodecyl sulfate are the common foaming agents present in many supermarket shampoos. These are the harmful agents which are harsh in nature. Frequent use of high concentration of sulfates has been linked to stripping away of natural moisture and hair protein. If you shampoo three times a week, use sulfate free shampoo at least one out of three times. Sulfates free shampoo strengthens your hair by preventing the damage.

4. Don't Stress Out

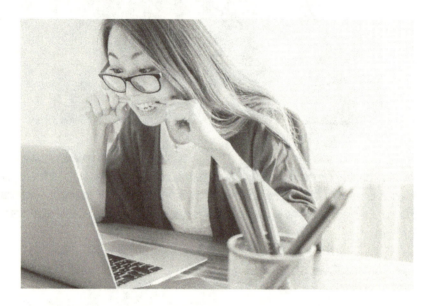

You must have noticed that you start losing your beautiful hair strands the moment you feel stressed. Relax! Nothing can be more dangerous than stress for your hair.

High-stress levels can result in three types of hair loss –

Telogen Effluvium – The stress pushes large numbers of hair follicles into a resting phase of the hair follicle (telogen phase), and your hair might fall out even when simply washing or combing your hair.

Alopecia Areata – When the immune system attacks hair follicles and the hair falls out in round patches.

Trichotillomania – When you can't resist an urge to pull out hair from your scalp. So, relax and let your hair live.

5. Oil Your Hair

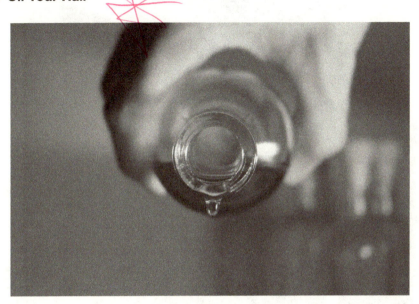

Nourish your hair frequently with natural oils. Take equal amount of coconut oil, olive oil, and almond oil and massage gently for 10–15 mins. Leave the oil overnight; so that, each strand soaks up the oil. Wash with shampoo and conditioner the very next day. If leaving overnight is not possible, you should leave the oil for at least 45 min, the longer you leave, the better will be the results. However, you should not leave it for more than 24 hours. Never go out with oiled hair as it attracts dirt, pollution and, grease that makes your hair weak and affect overall hair health.

6. Apply Henna Every Four to Six Weeks

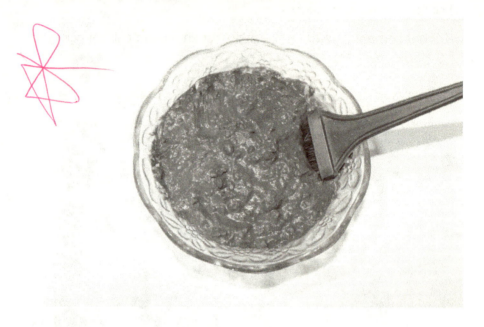

Henna (Mehndi) is a natural hair conditioner and natural hair dye. Henna is the best hair beauty secret that India has shared with the world. Benefits of henna are ample, it improves hair growth, prevents dandruff, reduces hair fall, and is a natural hair conditioner that gives deeply conditioned and nourished hair.

Make sure you check the label before buying the henna, it should contain 100% henna only without any other chemical agents such as chemical p-Phenylenediamine (PPD) which may irritate your scalp. Always try henna in a small portion on your skin, usually behind the ears to check any allergic reaction before fully applying on the head. Mix henna powder with water till it forms a thick paste. Now apply this paste to your hair. After an hour, rinse off with shampoo.

7. Rinse Your Hair with Diluted Vinegar

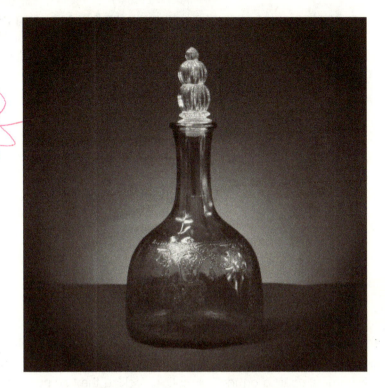

White or apple cider vinegar makes hair silky and shiny. Take one part of vinegar and two parts of water for normal type hair, rinse your hair with this mixture after shampoo. Wait for 5–8 mins then rinse with normal water. Your hair will be shinier and silkier than before — no need to condition your hair after shampooing if you are using a vinegar rinse.

If your hair is oily, then take an equal amount of vinegar and water. If your hair is dry, add a little more water. However, in any case, use diluted vinegar only, never use concentrated vinegar as it may dry out your hair and make it more prone to breakage.

8. Always Apply Conditioner After Shampoo

The primary function of the shampoo is to clean the hair, focussing mainly on the scalp. It removes any excess oil, grease, dirt or unwanted build-up. While cleaning, shampoo often dries the hair, making it frizzy, tangled, and hard to manage.

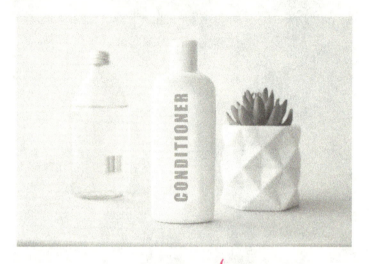

Untangling your hair may lead to hair fall. The conditioner works on hair strands, it forms a coating on the hair cuticle, locking the hair moisture and smoothen the hair, it protects hair from dirt and pollution, leaving a shiny finish.

9. Don't Sleep with Your Hair Tied Up

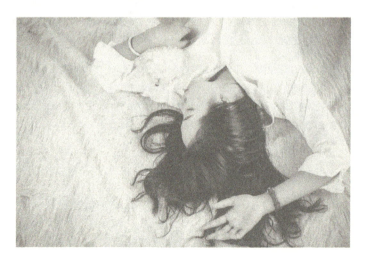

Sleeping with your hair tied up for almost 7–8 hours can put a strain on your scalp, weaken the roots which may lead to hair damage and hair fall. You may already know that body repairs when we sleep. When you are tieing your hair, you are preventing your hair from natural repair. So, don't put a strain on your scalp and let it breathe.

10. Eat Well

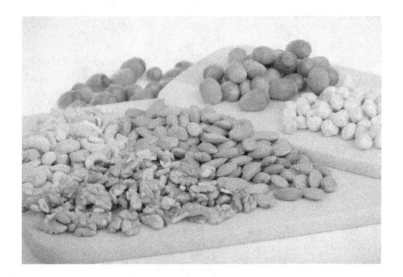

Hair gets profoundly affected by what you eat. Your diet should rich in protein, biotin, iron, and omega-3 fats. Protein promotes hair growth because hair follicles are made up of mostly protein called keratin. Biotin and iron prevent hair loss, and omega-3 fatty acids reduce inflammation, nourish your hair, and promote hair growth. If your diet is lack of these crucial nutrients, your hair health gets severely affected.

CONCLUSION

Your hair needs a little care and nourishment to look its best. Your eating habits and daily routine habits affect your hair health. Taking care of your hair inside out gives you the best results. Eating right nutrients and keeping your stress level to a minimum will internally nourish your hair while oiling your hair regularly and rinsing your hair with vinegar will protect your hair and give you shiny and healthy hair.

6
TOP 10 FOODS FOR SMOOTHER, SHINIER, STRONGER, AND HEALTHIER HAIR

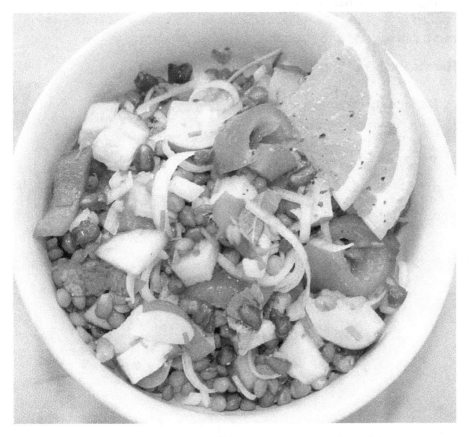

Top 10 Foods For Smoother, Shinier, Stronger, and Healthier Hair

There are so many hair care products available in the market. Also, they are being advertised in such a way that makes us think that our hair health and beauty is only and only depend on them. However, the reality is, they don't treat your hair problems; they just cover the flaws. No, doubt they can save you some time and give you a temporary solution. However, these products contain harsh chemicals which in long run can damage your hair and do more harm than good to your hair.

The only way by which you can have shinier, smoother, and healthier hair is by treating them internally. Your hair needs nutrition to work properly and to grow. Some foods are masters in doing that. These foods are packed with all the hair nutrients that can prevent split ends, tangles, dry, and brittle hair and give strength, volume, and shine to your hair.

Here is the list of Top 10 Foods for Healthier Hair:

1. Dark Leafy Greens

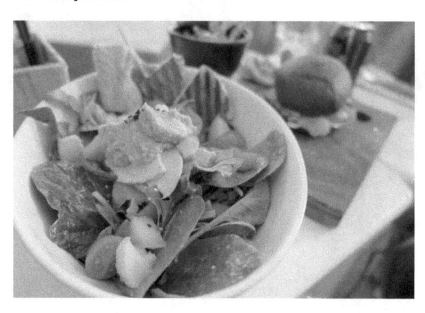

Dark leafy greens such as spinach, kale, fenugreek greens are excellent sources of iron, vitamin A, vitamin C, and calcium. Moreover, leafy greens are low in calories. Iron deficiency in the body means that the oxygen and essential nutrients are not reaching the roots and follicles of your hair, making the hair strands dull, and weaker. An iron deficiency can lead to hair fall, premature graying, and dull hair. To get full benefits of leafy greens don't boil them for too long, otherwise, you will lose out on the essential nutrients.

Best Way to Eat Leafy Greens: Cooking leafy greens can actually boost their antioxidant and iron content. You can grill or stir fry them. Always blanch before use but don't boil your leafy greens for a long time while blanching. Boiling in water causes a significant amount of nutrients like vitamin C, and folate to be leached away. A little salt in the water helps prevent all the nutrients coming out into the water.

Read 10 Power Foods To Get Rid Of Anemia in the previous book **Eat So What! The Power of Vegetarianism Volume 2 (Mini Edition).**

2. Nuts

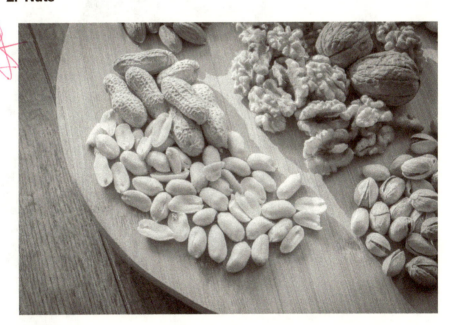

Omega-3 fats are essential nutrients and healthiest among other fats. Your body cannot produce them naturally, so you must get them from foods. Nuts are a great source of omega-3 fatty acids, which lubricate your hair strands, nourish your hair follicles and give thickness and shine to your hair.

Nuts such as almonds are also a great source of vitamin E that strengthen your hair, prevent dandruff and hair damage. Walnut oil contributes to the amount of elastin, a protein that is responsible for the elasticity in your hair strands hence prevent them from breaking. High beta-sitosterol content of pistachios has been proven to help with male-pattern baldness.

Nuts should be soaked in water overnight to lower its heat and phytic acid content, which reduces their health benefits.

3. Seeds

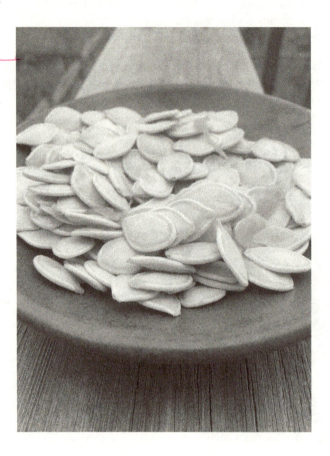

Seeds are not only a great source of omega-3 fatty acids but also a good source of zinc, magnesium, and antioxidants. Seeds are very low in calories that help keep your weight in check. Seeds such as flaxseeds, sesame seeds, and pumpkin seeds nourish the hair follicles and hair shafts, making them less prone to damage. They stimulate hair growth by conditioning and promoting a healthy scalp.

Hormone dihydrotestosterone (DHT) attaches to hair follicles and reduces anagen growth phase causing male pattern baldness. Beta-sitosterol of pumpkin seeds inhibits the 5-alpha-reductase enzyme that converts testosterone to dihydrotestosterone and prevents hair loss. Pumpkin seeds contain a good amount of zinc that prevents dandruff.

Flaxseeds lock moisture in your hair, making it smooth and manageable and prevent knotting and tangles. Flaxseeds are the richest dietary source of lignin, a potent antioxidant that helps in protecting hair cells from the aging process and prevent thinning of hair.

4. Citrus Fruits

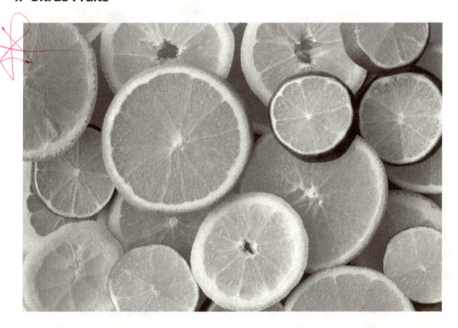

Citrus fruits are that category of fruits that are an excellent source of vitamin C. They strengthen the immune system and have anti-inflammatory and antioxidant effects. Why are citrus fruits important for hair? Because vitamin C increases the absorption of nonheme iron in your body. When you eat iron-rich food with vitamin C, it gives you the best results. Vitamin C helps in collagen production. Collagen is a type of protein that made up of amino-acids, proline, hydroxyproline, and glycine. Proline is also the main component of keratin, the type of protein that makes up your hair.

Some examples of citrus fruits are lemon, orange, and grapefruit. Add lemon juice when you blanch spinach, it will increase your iron absorption as well as prevent the spinach from losing its a dark green color.

Also, rather than have a glass of juice eat the whole fruit, since the fiber present in orange and grapefruit aids digestion.

5. Milk and Milk Products

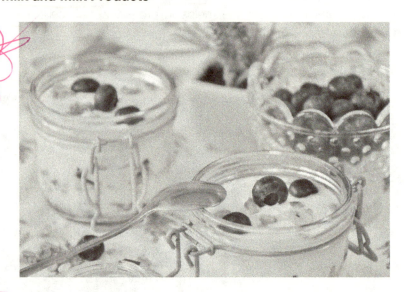

Every sip of milk does magic to your hair. Milk contains whey and casein, two important proteins for healthy hair. Having milk daily prevents hair loss and promotes hair growth and makes your hair stronger. Also, milk is an excellent source of vitamin B12. Deficiency in vitamin B12 can cause premature graying and can lead to anemia, which is a common cause of hair loss, tangles, and rough hair.

When applying topically, milk cream can be an excellent conditioner for your hair. It helps lock in the moisture and heal brittle, dry hair and split ends. Topical application of yogurt conditions the damaged and dry hair, making them smooth, shiny, and manageable.

Liquid whey, a by-product of cottage cheese-making, can stimulate hair follicles, strengthen the hair, help it grow faster and prevent the hair loss.

Milk and milk products are high in protein, vitamin D, and calcium. Go for skimmed milk and low-fat yogurt and cheese to cut back on some of the calories. Milk products work to restore natural luster and shine to the hair while strengthening its structure.

Eat Greek yogurt with honey, nuts, berries, and nuts for a delicious breakfast to give your hair complete nutrition.

6. Legumes

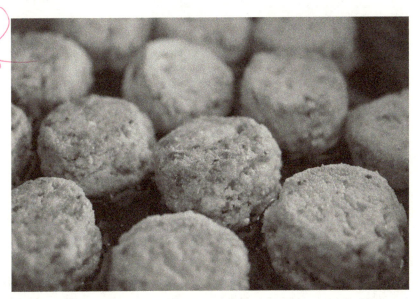

Legumes like lentils, chickpeas, kidney beans, peas, and peanuts are powerhouses packed with nutrients like protein, iron, folic acid, zinc, and biotin that support overall health wellness as well as your hair. Legumes contain essential vitamins and amino acids that are important for your hair health.

Lentils are rich in folic acid, which is essential for cell renewal and hair growth. Folic acid helps your body make red blood cells that supply scalp with much-needed oxygen.

Beans are a great source of protein, which is the building block of hair. Without enough protein, hair grows much slower, with weaker strands that are prone to breaking. Beans are a good source of zinc, which aids the hair growth and repair cycle and prevents dandruff.

Peas contain enough amount of vitamin C, which is involved in collagen formation, the hair follicles require collagen protein for optimal growth. Deficiency of vitamin C can lead to dry and brittle hair.

Falafel, enchiladas, or lentil soup with a fresh green leafy salad can be a good choice for your taste bud as well as for your hair.

7. Mung Bean Sprouts

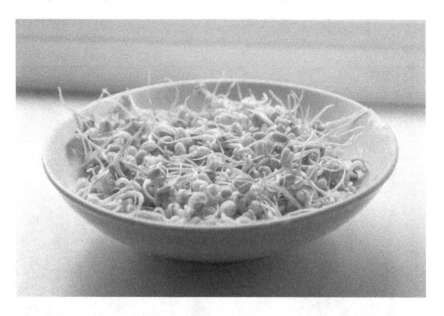

The practice of germinating seeds by which seeds or spores produce new leaves or buds called sprouting. Sprouting the beans increases their nutrient value, making beans richer in protein, iron, calcium, zinc, magnesium, phosphorus, and vitamins C content.

Sprouts have anti-bacterial and anti-fungal activities that help combat fungal growth that causes dandruff and other problems. They stimulate the production of sebum, the natural oil that helps keep the roots and hair strands moisturized and prevents split ends.

Sprouts contain enough vitamin C that strengthens the immune system; it destroys the free radicals in the body, which make the hair brittle. Vitamin C promotes hair growth.

The **sprouting process** starts with rinsing the beans with cold water. Place beans in a jar with water and soak them for 8–10 hours. Cover it with a mesh lid or muslin cloth, secure with a rubber band, to allow airflow. After 8–10 hours drain the water out through the muslin cloth. Give it a rinse with freshwater and drain again. Repeat this rinsing and draining process at least two to three time a day for the next three days and your nutritious sprouts are ready to eat. Eat them raw or sauté them with a little olive oil.

8. Mangoes

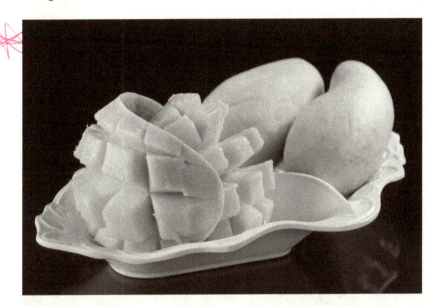

Beta-carotene is a bright reddish-orange pigment found in plants and fruits. It is beta-carotene that gives mangoes their vibrant yellow-orange color. It is known for its antioxidant property and high vitamin A activity. Body converts beta carotene into vitamin A.

Ripe mangoes hold large amounts of beta carotene, vitamin C and vitamin E, all of that have an antioxidant property that safely interacts with free radicals and neutralizes them to keep your hair healthy and strong. It prevents the hair follicle from shrinking and promotes hair growth.

If you have dull, lackluster hair, include Mangoes in your diet – it has scalp conditioning properties and gives your hair extra shine. Mangoes are a good source of vitamin A, which encourages the production of sebum, the natural oil that moisturizes your scalp to keep your hair healthy.

Vitamin C in mangoes promotes collagen production – the protein that provides the hair's elasticity and prevents it from breaking.

Mangoes are especially good for those with thinning hair because of the beta carotene. Thinning hair can be a sign of a vitamin A deficiency. Increasing Beta Carotene in your diet restores brittle, damaged hair, and promotes stronger, and healthier hair.

9. Sweet Potato

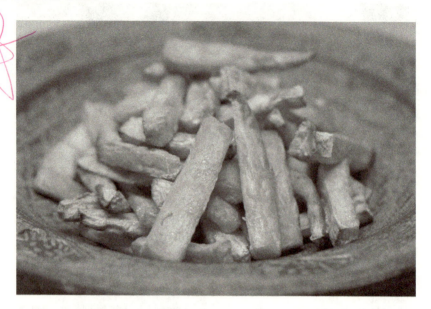

Sweet potato is a complete superfood for your hair that has almost all nutrients that your hair needs. It is low in calories and full of anti-inflammatory properties. It is high in beta carotene, Vitamin B6, C, D, and E and essential minerals like zinc, copper, iron, calcium, magnesium, and potassium.

Add sweet potatoes in your diet if you have a dry hair problem. Sweet potato provides massive nourishment to dry strands. Vitamin A will boost your scalp's natural oils, lock in the moisture, and promotes hair growth while the vitamin E adds shine by nourishing your hair follicles.

A deficiency in vitamin A can lead to dry, dull, and lifeless hair and leave your scalp itchy and lead to dandruff. Beta-carotene that is converted into vitamin A in our body is necessary for sebum production, and hair cell growth. However, don't overdo with vitamin A, excessive Vitamin A intake can have detrimental effects on the hair.

10. Water

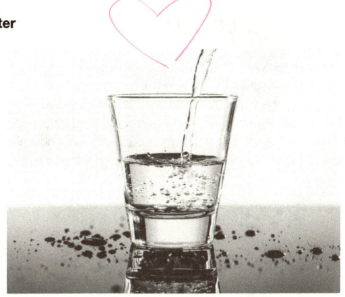

The list cannot be completed without the most crucial ingredient for your hair, that is water. Water is a key ingredient that delivers vitamins, and minerals to the hair which contribute to your hair growth.

You can intake all of the hair vitamins, protein, and minerals, but if you don't meet your body's daily water requirements, the nutrients will not reach the cells responsible for hair growth. As a result, cells will not be able to reproduce and grow, and your hair ends will split or become brittle. It is possible that dehydration can stop the natural growth cycle of your hair completely.

Just like plants, the root of the hair is the only means by which hair absorb the water and provide hydration to the hair, that naturally and internally boosts up hair growth.

Drinking at least two liters of water a day will not only keep your body healthy but also help to strengthen your hair follicles and promote hair growth.

CONCLUSION

Whatever you eat reflects on your hair. Give your body nutritious food; it will give you healthy hair in return. Similarly, giving junk foods to your body damage your hair and stunt their growth. If you want last longing permanent solution to your hair problems, include all foods as mentioned above in your diet. Moreover, these foods not only make your hair healthy but also give flawless, smooth, and soft skin and prevent aging of both your hair as well as your skin.

7
TOP 10 FOODS THAT PREVENT HAIR LOSS AND PROMOTE HAIR GROWTH

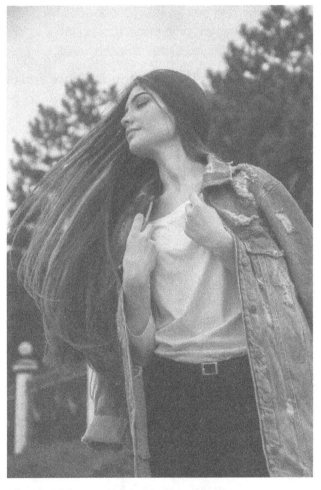

Top 10 Foods That Prevent Hair Loss and Promote Hair Growth

Before getting into the details of our super hair growth-promoting foods, one thing must be noted, hair loss or sudden drastic hair health changes can be an indication of an internal disease, like thyroid disease, lupus (an autoimmune condition), or a liver problem. Sudden shock or high-stress level can also lead to hair loss. It is normal to shed between 50 to 100 hairs a day, but if you experience massive hair fall, you need to consult a doctor to determine the underlying cause.

Most of the general causes of hair fall are nutritional deficiency and environmental damage. Fortunately, hair fall due to nutrition deficiency is reversible once you fulfill your hair nutrition requirement. Not only these foods prevent hair loss and but also are super effective in promoting the growth of new and healthy hair. With these superfoods, you can have long, strong, and healthier hair that you always wanted.

Below are the Top 10 Foods That Prevent Hair Loss and Promote the Rate of Hair Growth:

1. Amla/Indian Gooseberry

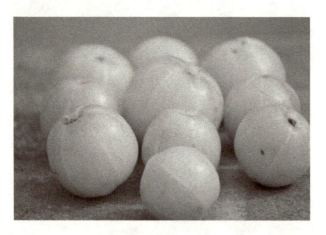

Amla also known as Indian gooseberry, the name amla itself means **amrit** or nectar, the drink of the gods. It is a sour fruit native to India. It is considered as anti-aging and natural tonic for hair as per Ayurved. This one single fruit contains billions of nutrients. Amla is one of the richest sources of vitamin C.

Along with vitamin C, amla is also extremely rich in antioxidants. Antioxidants neutralize the free radicals that can cause hair fall, and graying. Amla oil contains essential fatty acids that strengthen hair follicles and promote hair growth.

The phytonutrients, amino acids, vitamins, and minerals present in amla help to increase the scalp circulation, strengthen hair follicles, and stimulate healthy growth.

Vitamin C of amla increases collagen production. Collagen protein, the building blocks of hair, strengthens hair follicles that minimize the hair follicle damage and increases hair growth volume-wise as well as lengthwise.

2. Black Sesame Seeds

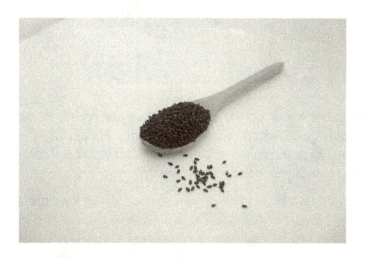

Black sesame seeds have the power to reverse graying & stimulate healthy hair growth. It promotes melanocyte cells to produce melanin – the pigment responsible for your hair color. Black sesame seeds contain essential fatty acids such as omega-3 that nourish, condition and promote a healthy scalp that stimulates healthy hair growth. Black sesame seeds are loaded with zinc, that helps in sebum production. This natural oil makes your hair shiny and lustrous.

Zinc also plays a role in the hair tissue repair and production of new hair cells. A deficiency in copper can lead to hair thinning and graying as copper play an important role in melanin production. Black sesame seeds are a good source of copper. Moreover, the high iron content of black sesame seeds prevents iron deficiency anemia, which is a common reason of hair fall.

3. Chia Seeds

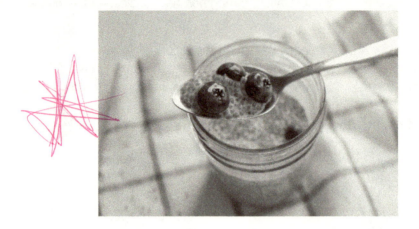

Chia seeds are full of potent nutrients. They are an excellent source of omega-3 fatty acids, which promote hair growth. Additionally, they are also a rich source of fiber, protein, and are full of antioxidants. It stimulates hair growth and makes your hair thick and healthy.

Moreover, iron, zinc, and calcium prevent further hair loss, make the scalp healthy, strengthen hair follicles, and ensure strong, thick, and healthy hair growth. A standard dosage recommendation of chia seeds is 15–20 grams (about 1.5 tablespoons). It should not be consumed in their dry, raw form. Soak chia seeds in water overnight and eat them in the morning or after work out.

4. Black Chickpeas (Kala Chana)

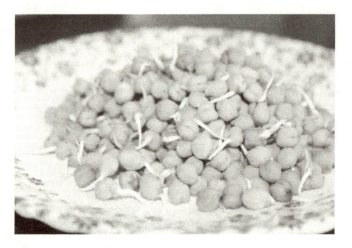

You must have heard lots of lecture from your mom on how Black chickpeas do a miracle to your hair, and she is not wrong. Black chickpeas indeed do magic to your hair. Every vitamin and mineral of black chickpeas contributes to hair growth as well as hair quality.

Black chickpeas are a great source of protein for vegetarians. Hair made up of mostly protein. Giving enough protein to your hair stimulates the growth of new healthy hair by strengthening your hair follicles; additionally, black chickpeas contain zinc and biotin. Both of these minerals improve your body's keratin infrastructure. Keratin is the structural protein which makes up the hair. Keratin is also the protein that protects scalp skin cells from damage or stress.

Vitamin A and iron in black chickpeas are crucial for hair health and deficiency in any one of these in the body can cause hair fall, brittle hair, and dandruff. Moreover, iron ensures the blood supply that contains important hair nutrient to the hair roots.

5. Raw Coconut

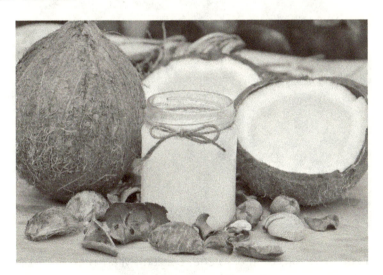

Fresh raw coconut at homes are quite common in India but finding it in western countries may be a little difficult but if you have access to raw coconuts include them in your diet as early as you can. Coconut cream, water, and oil are equally healthy. Coconuts are highly nutritious, rich in fiber, and packed with essential vitamins and minerals.

Lauric acid is the reason why coconut considers as a healthy fat even though it contains almost 89% of saturated fat. Lauric acid is a saturated fatty acid with a 12-carbon atom chain that has antibacterial, antiviral, and antimicrobial property; this potentially helps to prevent infections.

Coconut oil is good for your hair. Use coconut oil as a natural way to help your hair grow thicker, longer, and faster. The vitamins and essential fatty acids naturally found in coconut oil nourish the scalp and hair follicles.

Apply coconut oil mixed with olive oil and almond oil, a night before shampooing, massage gently and leave it overnight. Wash your hair with shampoo the very next day; it will help to heal your hair damage and naturally moisturize and treat split ends and frizzy hair.

6. Spinach

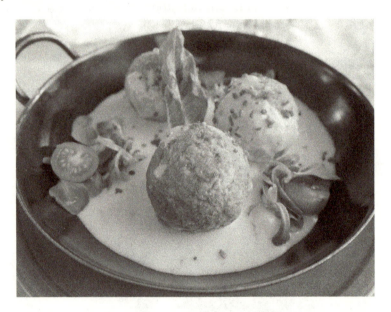

Spinach is rich in iron, beta-carotene, calcium, vitamin C, and fiber. These nutrients help nourish your scalp and hair, ensuring healthy hair growth. Regular consumption of spinach can prevent anemia and increase the supply of oxygen to the hair follicles, ensuring that they stay in top condition with all the right nutrients in them. Moreover, the anti-inflammatory properties of spinach help soothe an aggravated scalp.

Spinach is much better than red meat as it provides fewer calories and is fat and cholesterol-free. To make the most of its health benefits, include spinach in your daily diet. Make sure to combine vitamin-C-rich foods such as citrus fruits with spinach to improve absorption.

Pregnant women must eat spinach daily. Iron is imperative to healthy infant development, and the baby will have the healthiest hair. It also helps prevent severe defects of the brain in the baby.

7. Whole Grains

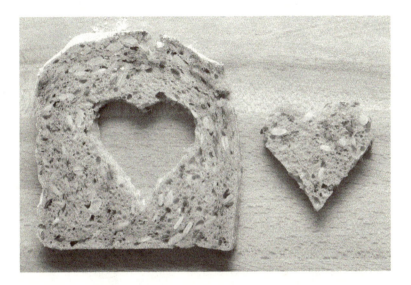

Whole grains, including brown rice and oats, are rich in biotin along with iron, B vitamins, and zinc. Biotin can help alleviate brittle hair and alopecia.

Biotin is required for cell proliferation; it also plays a vital role in producing a protein that breaks into amino acids in the body which are required for your hair to grow. Whole grains such as raw oats are also a good source of iron and zinc, the essential hair minerals. A deficiency in these minerals can lead to hair loss.

A combination of oats, milk, and almond oil is excellent for the hair. It can stop hair loss, stimulate hair growth, and adds shine to your hair strands. Next time when you plan to make a cake add whole wheat flour, oat flour (grind the oats), and semolina along with your regular flour, it will satiate your sweet craving also will nourish your hair.

8. Soybeans

Soybean is rich in high-quality protein, which your body uses to repair the cells and generate new tissue, including new hair. Additionally, soybeans are high in calcium, fiber, folic acid, iron, B vitamins, calcium, potassium, and fiber, which all are essential for healthy hair. Soybean oil reduces cellular damage and boosts new hair growth. Soybean oil is especially very beneficial for those suffering from hair loss problems.

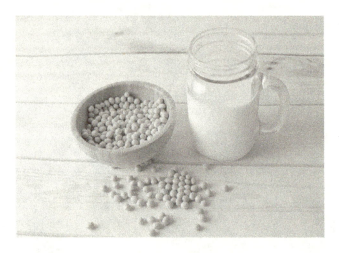

Soybeans are one of the richest food sources of spermidine, a polyamine. Spermidine stimulates hair-shaft elongation and prolongs the anagen (growth phase of hair), and thus directly promotes hair growth.

9. Carrots

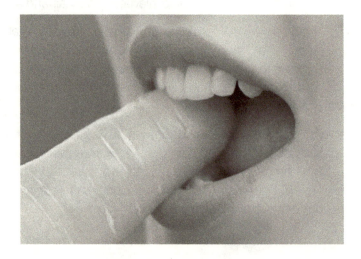

The vitamins A, B, C, E, phosphorus, and magnesium found in carrots improve the blood circulation in your scalp that ensures the reach of all other important nutrients to the hair root which in turn promotes hair growth.

These vital vitamins and minerals are effective in combating hair loss and protect your hair from turning dry and dull.

Carrots particularly loaded with beta-carotene, an antioxidant that converts to Vitamin A. This stimulates the sebaceous glands in the scalp to produce sebum that helps to keep your hair moisturized and make them thicker, shinier, stronger, and longer.

Drinking fresh carrot juice regularly can make your hair healthier and improve your eyesight.

10. Yogurt

Natural yogurt is full of protein, and vitamins that offer nourishment that your hair needs to grow strong and healthy. Yogurt has lactic acids, which relax and smooth the dry, scaly hair, and improve the natural moisture factor, making your hair more manageable. This is why you find lactic acids added in several shampoos and other hair products.

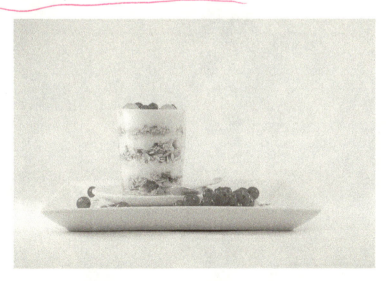

Yogurt is rich in vitamin B5, which enhances the blood flow to your scalp and promote hair growth. With its cooling effect, yogurt soothes an aggravated scalp. Its anti-fungal property helps to get rid of dandruff that soothes the scalp, improving scalp health and controls hair fall.

CONCLUSION

Healthy, silky, strong, and dense hair is everyone's goal. You don't need expensive hair treatments and fancy hair products to achieve this goal; the secret of long and healthy hair lies in your kitchen. Try adding above mentioned foods to your diet. These foods are rich in hair nutrients such as protein, B vitamins, vitamins A, C, D and E, zinc, iron, biotin, and essential fatty acids. Adding these nutrients to your diet may help treat hair loss and promote the hair growth rate.

2

HAIR PROBLEMS, THEIR REASONS, AND THEIR SOLUTIONS

1
HAIR PROBLEMS, THEIR REASONS, AND THEIR SOLUTIONS PART 1

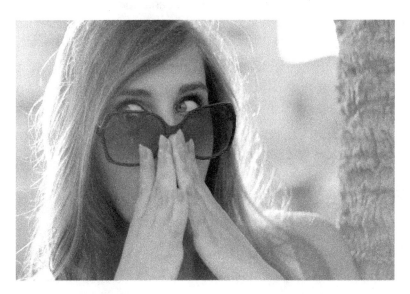

Hair Problems, Their Reasons, and Their Solutions Part 1

This chapter describes the following hair problems, their reasons, and their solutions:

- Gray/white hair
- Dandruff
- Frizzy hair
- Tangled hair

GRAY/WHITE HAIR

Melanocytes are cells in the hair bulb that produce melanin to provide your hair its natural color. Melanin production slows and finally stopped with age, which results in gray/white hair. But some people notice strands of white hair as early as in their teens which is commonly called premature graying.

Reasons for Premature Graying

1. Vitamin B12 deficiency can cause your hair to turn white prematurely (most common).

2. Hydrogen Peroxide is an oxidizing agent which is used for bleaching the hair. It penetrates the hair cortex and removes the natural pigment, melanin of the hair. Without melanin, the new hair grows without any pigment, and it appears gray or white.

3. Genetics play an important role in premature graying. If any of your parents became gray early, then most of the chances are that you may, too.

4. Smoking has long been linked to premature white hair. Toxins in cigarettes can damage your hair follicles, causing premature gray/white hair.

How to Treat White Hair Problem?

1. If you smoke, stop smoking as early as possible.

2. Don't color or bleach too often.

3. Eat food rich in antioxidant, and vitamin A. Studies suggest antioxidant, and vitamin A can boost your melanin production. Include carrots, sweet potatoes, and dark leafy vegetables in your diet.

4. White hair due to nutritional deficiencies can be revert with vitamin supplementation. Check your vitamin B12 level. A simple blood test can show whether your B12 levels are low. Don't be a doctor yourself and don't start taking supplements on your own instead concern your doctor for vitamin B12 supplements.

Read **Top 10 Foods For Vegetarians To Prevent Vitamin B12 Deficiency** in the previous book **Eat so what! The Power of Vegetarianism Volume 1 (Mini Edition).**

DANDRUFF

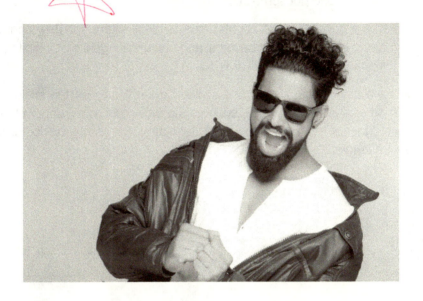

Dandruff is a condition of the scalp that involves itchy, scaly white flakes of dead skin cells. Dandruff is common in both men and women, all over the world.

Factors That Can Trigger Dandruff:

1. Over sebum secretions make skin oily and prone to dandruff.
2. A yeast called Malassezia is the metabolic by-products of skin micro-organisms that irritate the scalp and can cause more skin cells to grow.
3. Those who have high allergy sensitivity are more prone to dandruff.
4. Stress can trigger dandruff.

How to Treat and Prevent Dandruff?

1. Shampoo more often and use mild shampoo to avoid oil accumulation or any fungal infection.
2. Take diet rich in omega-3 fatty acids. They promote wound healing and help to manage oil production. Eat flaxseeds, nuts, and olive oil.

3. Don't stress out. Manage your stress level. Take a walk in the early morning and get some fresh air.

4. Use a good over the counter anti-dandruff shampoo. They contain zinc pyrithione, an antibacterial and antifungal agent that inhibits the fungal and bacterial cell division.

If you have severe dandruff or see scally fakes not only on the scalp but also on other areas of the body, such as the face, eyebrows, upper chest, and back, then it might be Seborrheic dermatitis. Concern your doctor for proper treatment.

SPLIT ENDS

When cuticle, the outmost protective layer of the hair shaft gets damaged, it splits from a single strand to two or multiple. The end is the most old, exposed, and vulnerable part of your hair; therefore, splits usually occur at the end. The damaged cuticle exposes the cortex, the main component of the hair; thus, hair becomes dull, weak and loses its texture and volume.

What Leads to Split Ends?

1. Over-Brushing

Brushing is good, it enhances blood supply to your hair, but over-brushing can do more harm than good. It compromises with your hair quality. It is advised to go easy with your hair.

2. Friction

If you are a long hair person and your hair brushes the back of your shirt, this friction may cause damage. Friction arises from towel can accelerate the development of split ends. Even fabrics of your scarves, sweaters, and hat can also lead to split ends.

3. Heat

Styling tools such as straighteners, blower, dryers, and curling rods induce high heat to the hair. Excessive heat may immensely damage your hair cuticles and cause split ends. It disturbs the moisture balance of the hair and leaves them dry, dull, and unhealthy.

4. Chemical Treatments

Chemical treatments such as hair colors and relaxers work in the cortex (inner, main layer of the hair) while damaging the protecting cuticle layer of your hair. Harmful chemicals present in them, damage the inner layer, thus resulting in split ends after a few weeks of treatment.

5. Excessive Use of Shampoo

Shampoo contains sulfates, the foaming agent that gives foam to the shampoo. The excessive use of sulfates can dry out your hair, and gives you split ends.

6. Alcohol

It is not only bad for your health but also make your hair worse. Alcohol dehydrates your hair, without optimum moisture, your hair becomes more prone to breaking and split ends. You might be thinking, why alcohol is added in some shampoos? Well, alcohol added in shampoos is different from drinking alcohol. Cetearyl alcohol and Cetyl alcohol are the common alcohol added in shampoos.

7. Poor diet

A diet lack in essential hair nutrients can cause your hair to dry. If your body is malnourished, your hair will be too, which make them more susceptible to split ends.

8. Environment

Excessive environmental exposures take a toll on your hair. Excessive exposure to sun and rainwater can accelerate the damage and results in split ends.

How to Prevent Split Ends:

1. Get a regular hair cut every 2–3 months or trim those split ends as you spot them; you'll catch the ends before they progress.
2. Use a mild shampoo that is SLS free.
3. Condition your hair post shampoo; it seals the cuticle.
4. Go easy with your hair while brushing.
5. Be gentle when you, detangle, style, and wash your hair.
6. Limit your alcohol consumption and drink plenty of water.
7. Eat plenty of leafy vegetables, nuts, beans, and carrots to nourish your hair internally.
8. Line your scarves and hats with silk to prevent any unwanted friction.

FRIZZY HAIR

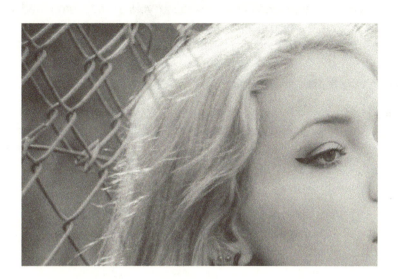

What Is Frizzy Hair?

If your hair does not align with other surrounding hair, instead it curls or stands up independently, creating an irregular swelled texture, then you have frizzy hair.

How Frizz Occurs?

Frizz occurs when the cuticle layer of your hair is damaged, moisture penetrates the hair shaft, absorbed into the cortex, and disturb the protein to moisture balance. As a result, hair appears swollen, frizzy, and dry instead of defined, silky, and smooth.

Another reason why your hair may appear Frizzy is due to a lack of moisture in the hair. To maintain the balance, your hair absorbs moisture from the air around it. This is the reason you get maximum frizz in the wet season.

Causes of Frizzy Hair:

1. Washing Your Hair with Hot Water.

Washing your hair with very hot water for a longer time can strip your hair off the natural oils that keep it moisturized, smooth and shiny.

2. Rough Brushing

Excessive or harsh brushing can cause your hair to stretched out of shape before it breaks, causing the remaining shorter hair to spring outward, away from the main body of hair.

3. Using Hot Tools on Wet Hair

Using hot tools like curling iron or straightener on wet hair can boil the water in the hair, causing bubbles to form inside the hair fiber which weakens the hair.

4. Over Shampooing

Washing your hair every day with shampoo is not healthy for your hair. The harsh foaming agents of shampoos can strip the hair of its natural oils resulting in dry, dull hair that looks frizzy.

5. Using Products with Too Much Protein

Giving too much protein to your hair without enough moisture can make your protein to moisture balance go off, which cause frizz.

6. You are Dehydrated

You aren't drinking enough water that is required to maintain optimum moisture in your hair.

7. Harsh Chemicals

Bleach and dye contain harsh chemicals that can damage the cuticle, the protective layer of the hair; as a result, moisture absorbs into the cortex, causing frizzy hair.

How to Prevent Frizzy Hair:

1. Don't use hot tools on wet hair. Keep their use to a minimum and always use them at their lowest temperature setting.
2. Drink plenty of water and eat a balanced diet.
3. Don't wash your hair every day.
4. Take a shorter shower with lukewarm water.

5. Avoid chemical over-processing on your hair.
6. Use Olive oil to oil your hair. It acts as an emollient and pulls moisture into the hair shaft. It is also good for hair growth.
7. Use a shampoo that contains dimethicone. It is a water-soluble, lightweight silicone that gives you silky and smooth hair. However, don't over depend on this for frizz hair as this gives you a temporary solution. You need to follow other above-specified remedies for a permanent solution.

TANGLED HAIR

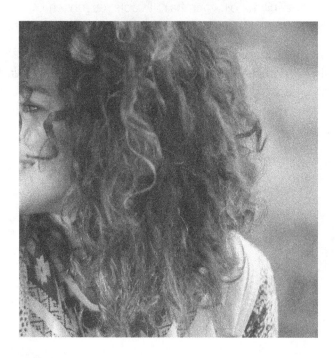

You are in a hurry in the morning, and it's getting late, you are all dress up, all you need to do is your hair but...but...but you can't comb through it. You are taking a small section of hair at a time but no, still can't comb through it. You waste your ample amount of time to detangle it, and again you are late today! Thanks to the tangled hair!! How many times have you experienced that?

Well, not anymore, there are some practical ways that you can use to stop your hair from getting tangled. But before we get into that, let's take a look at why you have tangled hair at the first place and what are the causes of hair tangling.

Why Hair Become Tangled?

It happens when the outer protective layer of your hair, the cuticle, becomes damaged. A healthy cuticle has a fish scale-like cells that overlap each other, they are smooth and closed, while a damaged cuticle has its layers open that become snagged on each other, resulting in tangles in your hair.

What Are the Causes of Tangled Hair?

1. Lack of Moisture

Absence of moisture in your hair can cause cuticle of your hair shaft break, which leads to friction and tension in your hair; as a result, you get a rough and damaged and tangled hair.

2. Not Combing Daily

If you don't comb every day, you are preventing your hair from nourishment. Combing activates the sebaceous gland, to produce sebum, the natural oil of the hair that keeps it moisturized.

3. Sleeping with Wet Hair

When you sleep with wet hair, the friction between your hair and the fabric of your pillow for 6–8 hours can cause your hair to tangle up.

4. Unhealthy Hair Ends

If your hair ends are dry, it can lead to split ends and frizz, which can tangle your hair easily.

5. Rough Towel Drying

When you rub your hair roughly and vigorously with a towel, it gives you a tangled mess.

6. Lack of Nutrition and Other Medical Condition

Sometimes iron deficiency, the buildup of ammonia in the body or hypothyroidism can lead to tangled hair.

How to Keep Your Hair Tangle Free

1. Use Conditioner After Shampoo

The best solution to prevent tangled hair is to use a conditioner after shampoo. It coats the hair strands and reduces friction between strands of hair, which in turn smoothens your hair and softens dry strands to allow easier brushing or combing. It locks the moisture as well as protect hair from dirt and pollution.

2. Nutrition Rich Foods

Eat plenty of almond, spinach, yogurt, and legumes. Eating food rich in iron and protein will sooth the cuticles and repair them faster.

3. Rinse with Cold Water After Shower

Washing your hair with hot water open up the cuticle layer. This is a simple yet effective step. Rinse your hair with cold water at the end of your shower; it will close your cuticles and prevent tangles.

4. Use a Silk Pillowcase

Just like your body needs rest, so do your sensitive tresses. Invest in a silk pillowcase as it does not cause friction and prevents your hair from getting tangled. Avoid cotton pillowcases; they are rough in texture that causes friction which can break your hair and cause tangles and knots in your hair.

5. Use a Wide-Toothed Comb

Brushing with a thin-toothed comb on tangled hair can lead to hair fall and further damage the hair as they can tear open the hair shafts. Also, it makes it quite challenging to detangle the hair with a thin-toothed comb. Instead, use a wide-toothed comb. Start at the ends and then work up to the roots. This way knot removes without pulling and damaging your hair too much.

Note

After you've tried these solutions, if your hair condition still doesn't improve or hair problem occurs with weakness, fatigue, massive hair loss or intolerance to cold, see your doctor to determine the underlying cause and to make sure you don't have a health problem.

2
HAIR PROBLEMS, THEIR REASONS, AND THEIR SOLUTIONS PART 2

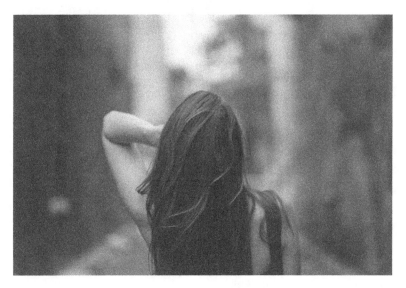

Hair Problems, Their Reasons, and Their Solutions Part 2

This chapter describes the following Hair problems, their reasons, and their solutions:

- Hair Fall
- Greasy Hair
- Dry Hair
- Head Lice

HAIR FALL

Losing between 50 and 100 hairs a day is completely normal. Hair fall problem is not life-threatening, but it severely hurt one's self-confidence by drastically changing the way he/she looks. Men, women, and even children can experience hair loss. This condition generally occurs as a result of hormonal changes, heredity, medical conditions, or as a side-effect of some medications.

Hair loss can be temporary or permanent. About 90 to 95% of the hair follicles are normally in the growth phase and replace the lost hair, but this doesn't always happen. Some factors affect the hair growth cycle and stunt its growth.

If you experience massive hair fall all sudden, you should consult with your doctor to diagnose the underlying cause of your hair loss and for appropriate treatment plans.

Factors That Lead to Hair Loss:

1. Stress

Stress is one of the major reasons for hair loss, hair thinning, and balding. Stress can push your hair follicles into a resting phase, and they don't produce new hair strands.

2. Lack of Nutrition

A diet lacking in protein, iron, and other B vitamins can lead to hair fall.

3. Medications

Certain medications that are used to treat depression, blood pressure, and heart problems or chemotherapy commonly cause hair loss.

4. Sudden or Extreme Weight Loss

Sudden change in the body mass index causes physical stress, which signals the hair follicles to move into telogen phase (resting phase).

5. Genetics

If your mom or dad has a hair loss problem, then there are fair chances that you may too have this problem.

6. Hormonal Changes

Hormonal changes like those in puberty, pregnancy, and menopause may cause hair loss.

7. Aging

It is normal to get thinning hair as you age, for both men and women.

8. Trauma

Hair loss can happen after a shock or a traumatic event such as losing the job or surgery.

9. Certain Diseases or Medical Conditions

Hair loss can be a result of an underlying illness, such as hypothyroidism, liver disease, and systemic lupus erythematosus.

Hair Loss Types:

Alopecia Areata: It is a common autoimmune disorder in which the immune system attacks the hair follicles, resulting in hair loss, usually in round patches. The hair often grows back within a year.

Traction Alopecia: This gradual hair loss, caused primarily by persistent pulling or traction on hair roots. This commonly results from tight ponytails and braids that pull hard enough the hair to make it fall out.

Male Pattern baldness: This is the most common type of hair loss in men. It usually begins at the temples or the crown of the head.

Female Pattern Baldness: In women, thinning often starts as a widening of the center hair part, with a preserved hairline but hair loss rarely proceeds to baldness as in men.

Postpartum Alopecia: Hormones fluctuate during pregnancy, and hair become fuller and thicker. However, women experience hair loss after delivering a baby that eventually normalize without treatment.

Trichotillomania or Trich: Trich is characterizing as an irresistible urge to pull out one's hair. Hair pulling cause patches of noticeable hair loss.

Telogen Effluvium: A reversible condition in which hair falls out after a stressful shock such as surgery, hair can abruptly fall out in large patches resulting from the early entry of hair in the resting phase. Typically, hair often grows back when the stress goes away.

Tinea Capitis (Ringworm): A fungal infection of the scalp caused by fungi called dermatophytes, creates round patches of itchy, scaly skin with hair loss. There is not really a worm involved in tinea capitis; it is called so because spots appear in a ring shape.

How to Treat and Prevent Hair Fall:

1. Maintain a good hair hygiene with regular shampooing, at least 2–3 times a week depending upon your hair type.
2. Get your CBC (complete blood count) done, CBS is a blood test used to evaluate underlying medical conditions like thyroid disease, and anemia.
3. Include food rich in iron and vitamin B, in your diet to promote hair growth.
4. Massage your scalp with hot oil (coconut oil, almond oil, and olive oil) using your fingertips. It increases the flow of the blood circulation to the hair follicles, conditions your scalp, and promotes hair growth.
5. Avoid hair treatments like coloring, and straightening as much as you can.
6. Limit your heating tools usage. If you really need to use, keep it on the lowest heat setting.
7. Apply aloe vera to your hair and scalp, leave it for about 45 minutes and rinse with normal water. Do this at least two times a week for better result.

HEAD LICE

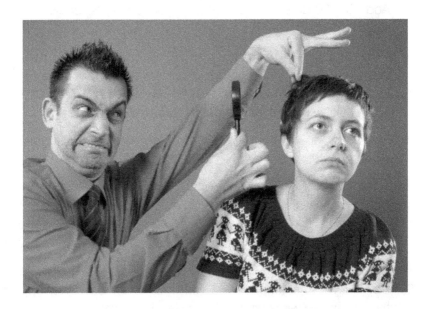

Head lice infestation and nits are the infections of the head hair by the head louse. They are about the size of a sesame seed and can be brown, dark gray or white. Head-lice infestations are common, especially in children. They are spread by direct contact with the hair of someone infected. Itching from lice bites is common.

Head lice are only able to survive on human head hair as they only feed on human blood. Without the human host, they are unable to live beyond three days. Head lice are not known to spread any disease. During a person's first infection, the itch may not develop for up to six weeks.

Causes of Lice:

1. It spreads through head-to-head contact with the hair of an infected person.
2. By sharing head-touching items such as combs, hats, scarves, towels, and earbuds.

How to Prevent and Get Rid of Head Lice?

1. Add 15 – 20 drops of Tea tree oil in your shampoo bottle. It repels lice.

2. Oil your hair with warm coconut oil and neem oil and massage gently. Both oils have antibiotic properties and known to deter lice. Use the nit comb to work through the oil-treated hair. Oil makes nits activity slower, and they come out much more easily.

3. Head lice dislike the smell of the essential oils like menthol, eucalyptus oil, lavender oil, and rosemary oil. Most likely, lice hate the smell of these strong oils.

4. Use an essential oil spray. Take 30 ml of water and add 5–6 drops of essential oil in it. Fill this solution in a spray bottle. Essential oils such as peppermint, eucalyptus, lavender, and rosemary cause the nits to loosen more easily.

5. Buy lice killing shampoo from your local pharmacy. After applying the shampoo, wrap your hair with a plastic bag and let it sit for half an hour, it stuns lice. Afterward, comb out the lice and eggs with a nit comb and take a shower, rinsing all the shampoo out. Finally, clean the Combs in the boiling water, while washing clothes, bedsheets, and pillow-covers in hot water. With proper care, you can prevent them from recurring.

GREASY HAIR

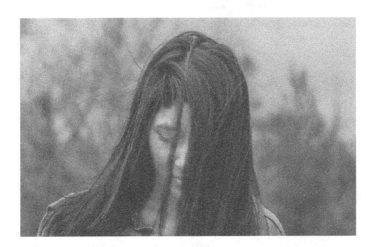

Overactive sebaceous glands are the reason behind your oily hair. Sebaceous glands make sebum, the natural oil that keeps the hair smooth, healthy, and prevents it from drying out and breaking. However, too much sebum can cause the hair to look greasy. An excessively oily scalp is related to outbreaks of dandruff.

What Causes Oily Hair?

1. Touching Your Hair

Touching your hair too much can transfer the oil from your hands to your hair, making it greasy.

2. Brushing Too Much

When you brush your hair, it increases blood flow to the hair follicle, but it also stimulates sebaceous glands to produce more sebum, which leads to oily hair.

3. Unhealthy Eating Habits

What you eat affects your hair health. When you eat foods that are high in saturated fats, they lead to greasy hair.

4. Climate

The region where you live can be another contributing factor to greasy hair. Sebaceous glands become overactive in warmer weather. High levels of humidity can also lead to a greasy scalp.

5. Hormonal Changes

Some girls may experience greasy hair during the first days of the period. The sebum production is actually increased before menstruation due to an increase in the hormone called androgens. This could be the probable cause of your greasy hair.

6. Your Shampoo Might have Oil in it

Some shampoos contain natural oils such as olive oil for silky and shiny hair, but if you have already oily hair, this can make your hair even more greasy. Check the label before buying your shampoo.

How to Prevent Greasy Hair?

1. Avoid eating foods that are high in saturated fat.
2. Add vitamin B2 and B7 rich foods to your diet. It helps moderate your sebum production.
3. Don't oil your hair too often, limit it to once a week.
4. Wash your hair at least 2–3 times a week.
5. Use shampoo and conditioner specially made for greasy hair that doesn't contain any oil.
6. Rinse your hair with diluted Apple cider vinegar at the end of your shower. It will help to restore the pH balance of your scalp and control sebum production.
7. Talcum powder and other powders are also useful in absorbing grease, but this a last-minute save for your greasy hair. Wash your hair with shampoo as early as you can otherwise it will lead to buildup on your scalp.

DRY HAIR

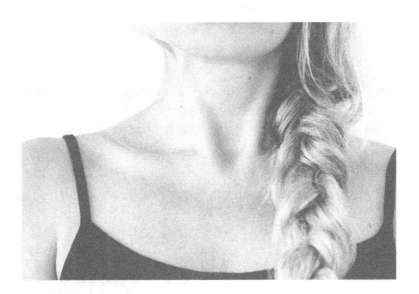

Why Hair Gets Dry?

Hair gets dry when it doesn't have enough moisture. Sometimes, sebaceous glands in scalp don't make enough sebum, the natural oil that lubricates hair and keeps your hair moisturized and looks lustrous. Because hair doesn't have enough oil, it looks dry.

The damaged cuticle layer of the hair can also lead to dry hair. The cuticle is the outermost protective layer of the hair. It protects hair from environmental pollution, dirt and sun damage; it also helps to lock in moisture in the hair. When this layer got damaged, it loses its close structure and let some oil escape and hair becomes dry.

What Factors Lead to Dry Hair?

1. Genetics

Sometimes it's not your fault that your hair is dry. Neither any of your habits nor any chemicals are responsible for dry hair. It is because you inherited it from your parents. If any of your parents or both have dry hair, it is most likely that you will also have dry hair.

2. Over-Washing

Washing your hair is a healthy habit, but overdoing may strip away your hair's natural oils.

3. Heavy Chemical Shampoo

In order to give good looks to your hair, shampoo making companies sometimes add a lot of chemicals which provide a good cover to your hair flaw, but in the long run, it damages the hair and makes it dry.

4. Environmental Pollution

When you expose your hair to lots of dirt, pollution or sun, it leads to dry hair.

5. Hot Tools

Using curling irons, hair straighteners or blow-drying your hair too often damage the cuticle which leads to moisture escape from hair.

6. Overuse of Alcohol-Based Products

Excessive use of alcohol-based styling products dehydrate the hair.

How to Prevent and Treat Dry Hair?

1. If you have dry hair, limit your hair wash to once or twice a week.
2. Massage coconut oil into your scalp before shampoo and leave for at least 45 mins to replenish moisture.
3. Either use a natural shampoo with least chemicals or dilute your shampoo before using. Take about half amount of shampoo that you usually apply and dilute it with about one-fourth cup to water. Make foam in it with your hands and use this diluted shampoo in place of your regular shampoo.
4. Follow the shampoo with a conditioner that contains argan oil and olive oil. It will keep the cuticles close, so they hold in natural oils.
5. Use hair products that don't contain alcohol.

Note

After you've tried these solutions, if your hair condition still doesn't improve or hair problem occurs with weakness, fatigue, massive hair loss or intolerance to cold, see your doctor to determine the underlying cause and to make sure you don't have a health problem.

3

DIET PLAN & LIFESTYLE GUIDE SEASON WISE

WINTER, SUMMER & MONSOON

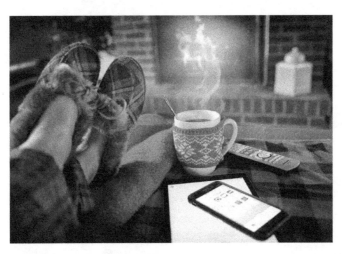

Diet Plan & Lifestyle Guide Season Wise: Winter, Summer & Monsoon

WINTER

The cold air of this season can dry out your hair and scalp.

LIFESTYLE GUIDE

1. Drink plenty of water to prevent your hair and scalp from dehydration.
2. Wear a hat while stepping outside. Make sure it's not too tight that it restricts the circulation in your scalp and causes hair fall.
3. Oil your scalp and hair regularly. During the winter season, your scalp will be drier, which forces sebaceous glands to make even more sebum, and that can lead to scalp irritation and dandruff.
4. Wash your hair with warm water. Make sure water is not too hot or else it will strip off the natural oils from the hair.
5. You may increase the amount of your conditioner after shampoo if you find your hair is becoming too dry.
6. Don't go out with wet hair. Cold weather can make your hair dry by absorbing the moisture. Let it dry naturally before going outside.

DIET PLAN

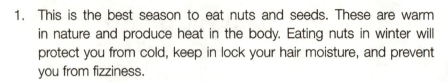

1. This is the best season to eat nuts and seeds. These are warm in nature and produce heat in the body. Eating nuts in winter will protect you from cold, keep in lock your hair moisture, and prevent you from fizziness.

2. Eat soaked 8 almonds, 2 walnuts, 8 pistachios, and 5 cashew nuts daily. If you are keeping a watch on your weight, eat them every alternate day, or reduce the quantity.

3. Winter is the season of green leafy vegetables. Eat plenty of spinach, fenugreek leaves, Bathua (Chenopodium album).

4. Eat more colorful fruits and veggies this season, including carrots and sweet potatoes.

SUMMER

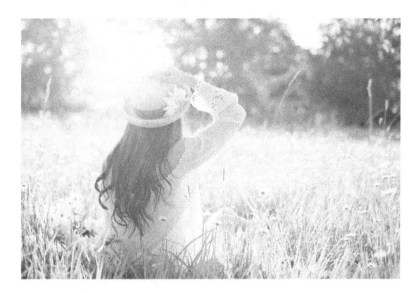

Summer is a season of greasy hair and irritated scalp.

LIFESTYLE GUIDE

1. Avoid going out between 1 pm to 4 pm.
2. Cover your hair with cap, or stoles, when stepping out.
3. Use conditioner containing SPF protection to protect your strands from harsh UV rays.
4. Summer is the season of excessive perspiration. Drink plenty of water to remove toxins from the body. Drink plain lemon water (without sugar or salt) after waking up.
5. Wash your hair regularly.
6. Maintain good hair hygiene.
7. Apply henna on your hair. This will keep your scalp in more cooling condition as well as nourish your hair.

DIET PLAN

1. Drink lemon water every day.
2. Eat sprouts such as mung bean, black chickpeas, and whole grains sprouts.
3. This is the season of mangoes. Eat up to 3 mangoes in a day. Limit the quantity to one if you are on your weight loss mission.
4. Include yogurt in your diet. Add chia seed in your yogurt. Make sure to soak chia seeds before using them.
5. Eat grapes and pineapple for your healthy and faster hair growth.

MONSOON

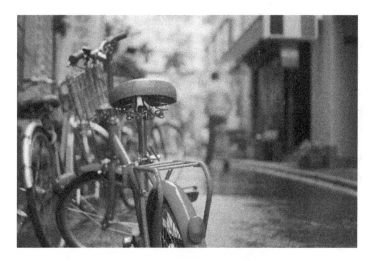

This season can increase your fungal infection due to high moisture in the atmosphere.

LIFESTYLE GUIDE

1. Rainwater is often loaded with pollutants. Shampoo your hair 2–3 times a week to remove any dirt and contaminant from your hair.//
2. Conditioner is a must in this season. Use a conditioner containing olive oil and argan oil every time you shampoo your hair.
3. Oil your hair regularly but don't keep it for long, it can irritate your scalp.
4. Use hair products that don't contain alcohol.
5. Rinse your hair with diluted Apple cider vinegar at the end of your shower. It will give shine to your frizzy hair.
6. Trim your ends. If you see any damage to your hair ends, get them trimmed. If you don't cut those ends, they will split all the way up the hair shaft, causing more damage to your hair.

DIET PLAN

1. Hair gets easily damaged in the wet season. Eat plenty of protein in this season. Protein will strengthen your hair follicles and make them strong and unbreakable.

2. Eat soybeans and soy products like tofu, soy milk.

3. Include blueberries in your diet. Blueberries facilitate Hair Growth and prevent premature graying.

4. Eat guava and guava leaves. Guava leaves contain vitamin C, which helps boost collagen activity that helps hair grow out faster and healthier.

5. Include lots of almonds, walnuts, and dates in your diet. These are rich sources of essential fat and antioxidants, that boost hair growth.

4

RECIPES

THAT PROMOTE HAIR HEALTH AND GROWTH

BEAN SALAD

(La Fonceur Original Recipe)

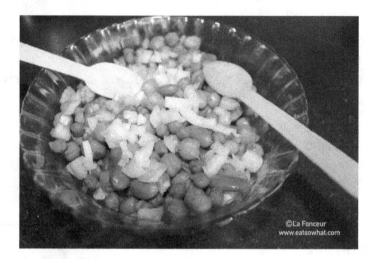

Ingredients:

Chickpeas/Garbanzo beans – 75 gm

Black chickpeas – 75 gm

Kidney beans – 75 gm

Peanuts – ½ cup

Onion – 1 medium

Soy sauce – 3 tablespoons

Crushed black pepper – a pinch

Salt – To taste

Dried mango powder (Amchoor) – ½ teaspoon

Method:

1. Wash chickpeas, kidney beans, and black chickpeas separately. Soak them in warm water for about 8–10 hours.
2. After 8–10 hours, they will be double in size. Wash them with fresh water.
3. Soak the peanuts in water for 2 hours. Soaked peanuts give an amazing taste.
4. Now take a pressure cooker, add all the soaked ingredients, add about 1 cup of water and a pinch of salt. Close the lid and cook till they tender. Don't overcook them. Turn off the flame after three whistles.
5. Once chickpeas, kidney beans, and black chickpeas, and peanuts are cooked, take them in a bowl, remove any excess water. Add salt (remember you have added salt while boiling too, so watch the quantity), soy sauce, black pepper, dried mango powder. Let them marinate for 4–5 hours.
6. Now add finely chopped onion, and it's ready to eat.

Nutrition Facts

Beans (Black Chickpeas, Garbanzo Beans, Kidney Beans): Beans are a great source of protein, which is the building block of hair. Without enough protein, hair grows much slower, with weaker strands that are prone to breaking. Beans are a good source of zinc, which aids the hair growth and repair cycle and prevent dandruff.

Peanuts: Peanuts are full of biotin that promotes hair growth and overall scalp health. A deficiency can cause brittle hair. The amino acids and protein present in peanuts help healthy hair growth. Peanuts have a warm nature and produce heat in the body. Soaking peanuts before use can decrease its heat.

Onion: Onion contains sulfur that helps reduce breakage and thinning of hair. Sulfur is essential for regeneration of hair follicles. The onion improves blood circulation in the scalp, promoting hair growth.

Black Pepper: Black pepper is rich in Vitamins A, iron, and antioxidants such as flavonoids, and carotenoids. These Essential nutrients in black pepper provide strengthening and protecting effect on the hair.

CRUNCHY CHOCOLATE OATS DROPS

(La Fonceur Original Recipe)

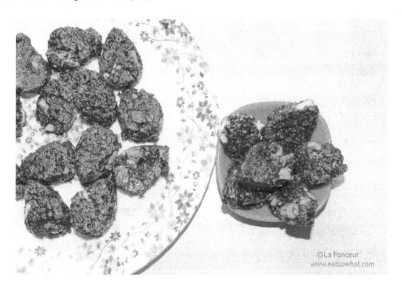

Ingredients:

Dark chocolate compound – 100 gm

Oats – 1 cup

Chopped Almonds – ¼ cup

Chopped Walnuts – ¼ cup

Marie biscuit – 3

Milk powder – 15 gm

Milk – 50 ml

*Cup size in this recipe – 200 ml cup

Method:

1. Heat a pot with several inches of water and place another bowl with chocolate inside over it.
2. Stir occasionally and allow the chocolate to melt in the bowl.
3. Once the chocolate is completely melted remove it from heat.
4. Add milk powder and milk into it and continue to stir until it reaches a smooth consistency. Keep it aside to let it cool for some minutes.
5. Now take a thick bottom pan. Heat it. Once hot, bring the flame to medium and add oats, almonds, and walnuts. Stir slowly. Keep stirring otherwise oats will start burning. After two minutes, add pieces of Marie biscuits in the pan.
6. Roast till it gives out a pleasant aroma and starts turning a bit brown. Turn off the flame and keep the pan aside. Let it cool.
7. Once the mix cools, add roasted oats, almonds, walnuts, and biscuits in melted chocolate, mix them well. Chocolate must coat all the ingredients thoroughly.
8. Pour this mixture in a plate and flatten it with the use of spatula. Cut in the desired shape with a cookie cutter while it is still hot.
9. Refrigerate for 2 hours and yummy crunchy chocolate oats drops are ready to eat.

Tips: Never try to melt chocolate on direct flame; it will burn the chocolate. Always use a double boiler.

* Dark chocolate compound already contain sugar so no need to add more sugar.

* Don't add oats mixture in the melted chocolate while it is still hot. Oats will turn soggy, and it will lose its crunchiness.

Nutrition Facts

Oats: Oats are a gluten-free whole grain and a great source of essential vitamins, minerals, fiber, and antioxidants. Oats are a good source of iron and zinc the essential hair minerals. A deficiency in these minerals can lead to hair loss.

Almonds & Walnuts: Almonds are a great source of vitamin E that strengthen your hair, prevent dandruff and hair damage. Walnut oil contributes to the amount of elastin, a protein that is responsible for the elasticity in your hair hence prevent them from breaking. Nuts are a great source of omega-3 fatty acids, which provide lubrication and nourishes your hair and gives thickness and shine to your hair.

Dark Chocolate: Dark chocolate is full of copper, zinc, and iron. These minerals promote the cell renewal growth process and healthy hair growth. Dark chocolate is a rich source of antioxidants that fight free radicles in the body and slow down the aging process of hair.

Milk & Milk Powder: Milk and milk products are high in protein, vitamin D, and calcium. Also, milk is an excellent source of vitamin B12. Deficiency in vitamin B12 can cause premature graying and can lead to anemia, which is a common cause of hair loss, tangles, and rough hair.

PALAK PANEER

(Cottage Cheese In Spinach Gravy)

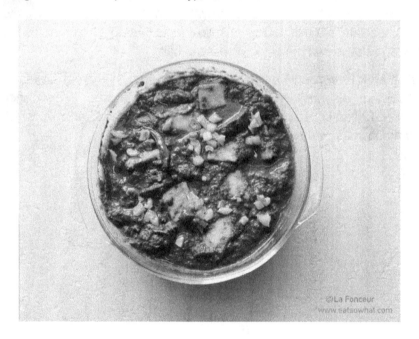

Ingredients
For Spinach Paste:

    Fresh spinach – 250 gm (about 2 cups)

    Ginger – 1 inch

    Garlic – 2 cloves

    Green chili – 3

    Lemon juice – 1 tablespoons

    Water – 5 cups

Other Ingredients:

Cottage cheese cubes – 10 to 12

Onion paste – 1 cup

Tomato puree – ½ cup

Salt – To taste

Ghee (Clarified butter)/butter – 2 tablespoons

Groundnut oil – 2 tablespoons

Red chili powder – 1 teaspoon or as per taste

Grated ginger – 1 tablespoon

Chopped garlic – 2 tablespoons

Garam masala – 1 tablespoon

Clove – 2

Bay leaf – 1

Water – ¼ cup, if required

Method

1. Bring a large pot of water to boil. Add the fresh spinach, submerge them in the water. Add a pinch of salt and lemon juice.
2. Blanch until the spinach leaves are no longer rigid (about 1 mins) and then drain the spinach and dump into a bowl of cold water to prevent it from losing its dark green color. Leave it for 5 min.
3. Take out the spinach.
4. Take blanched spinach, ginger, garlic, and green chili and blend to smooth paste without adding any water. Keep this paste aside.
5. Heat 1 tablespoon of oil in a pan and stir fry cottage cheese until golden brown.
6. Remove the cottage cheese. Add another tablespoon of oil and add cumin, when it splutters, add bay leaf and cloves.

7. When it starts to crackle add ginger, garlic and cook till it turns a little brown.
8. Add onion paste. Cook about 5–7 mins on medium flame till it leaves oil.
9. Add tomato puree and cook for another 5 mins.
10. Add garam masala, red chili powder, and salt. Cook for 3 mins on medium flame.
11. Add prepared spinach paste and cook for 5 minutes. Don't overcook; spinach will be decolorized.
12. Now add cottage cheese cubes to the mix and simmer till they absorb flavor.
13. Turn off the flame and add 2 tbsp of hot ghee or butter whichever is available with you, mix well and serve hot.
14. Eat palak paneer with chapatti, naan or brown rice.

Nutrition facts

Spinach: Spinach is rich in iron, beta-carotene, calcium, vitamin B9, and C and fiber. These nutrients help nourish your scalp and hair, ensuring healthy hair growth. Regular consumption of spinach can prevent anemia and increase the supply of oxygen to the hair follicles, ensuring that they stay in top condition with all the right nutrients in them.

Cottage Cheese: Cottage cheese is rich in protein. Inadequate protein intake can cause hair to fall. Protein provides strength to the hair shaft and reduces the chances of hair fall by breaking and splitting. Also, cottage cheese is an excellent source of vitamin B12 that prevent premature graying and hair fall.

Mushroom: Mushroom contains selenium that is vital for healthy hair. Selenium compounds can kill Malassezia, a fungus present on the scalp and are responsible for causing dandruff. Mushrooms also contain high levels of iron and copper. Iron prevents anemia, and copper facilitates the absorption of iron from food, promoting strong and healthy hair.

Onion: Onion contains sulfur that helps reduce breakage and thinning of hair. Sulfur is essential for regeneration of hair follicles. The onion improves blood circulation in the scalp, promoting hair growth.

Tomato: Tomatoes are a rich source of vitamin C which promote hair growth. Additionally, tomatoes contain Vitamin A, B, and E, which help prevent hair loss, give natural silk and shine and help treat dandruff.

Spices: Herbs and spices are not only good for hair but also for overall health. Spices increase blood flow to the hair follicle, and the blood delivers essential nutrients for faster and healthier hair growth.

SESAME, PEANUT, AND COCONUT CHIKKI

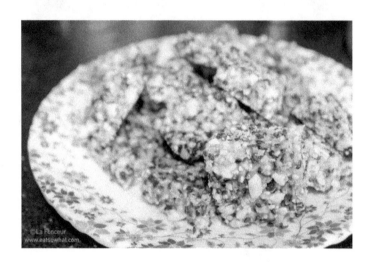

Ingredient

Black sesame seeds – ½ Cup

White sesame seeds – ½ Cup

Roasted peanuts – 1 Cup

Roasted desiccated coconut – 1 Cup

Jaggery/Panela – 3 Cup

Method

1. Dry roast each of the ingredient except jaggery individually till it gives an aroma and turns to a little brown.
2. Remove the outer layer of peanuts. Rub peanuts in between your hands to remove the outer skin. Crush them coarsely with the help of a chopper.

3. In a heavy-bottomed pan, add jaggery. Put the flame on medium and let it melt completely.

4. Once all the jaggery has melted, cook for no more than 2 mins on medium flame.

5. Bring the flame to low and add crushed peanuts, roasted black, and white sesame seeds and roasted desiccated coconut into melted jaggery. Mix well until all ingredients combined. Turn off the flame.

6. Now spread the mixture on a greased plate. Cover it with a wax paper. Use a rolling pin to spread it evenly. Let it cool completely.

7. After 5 minutes, use a sharp knife to cut them in squares or any of your desired shape and enjoy sesame, peanuts and coconut chikki.

Tips: Roasting all the ingredients is an important step as roasting enhance their taste.

* Don't overcook jaggery, it will make your chikki super hard and impossible to chew. We need our chikki to be firm and chewy.

* We are adding white sesame seeds along with black sesame seeds because black sesame seeds alone can have a very strong taste. It can even give a bitter taste. If you are okay with a little bitterness, replace the ½ Cup of white sesame seeds with another ½ Cup of black sesame seeds.

Nutrition Facts

Sesame Seeds: Sesame seeds have the power to reverse graying & stimulate healthy hair growth. It promotes melanocyte cells to produce melanin – the pigment responsible for your hair color. Black sesame seeds contain essential fatty acids such as omega-3 that nourish, condition and promote a healthy scalp that stimulates healthy hair growth.

Peanuts: Peanuts are full of biotin that promotes hair growth and overall scalp health. A deficiency can cause brittle hair. The amino acids and protein present in peanuts help healthy hair growth.

Desiccated Coconut: Coconut is good for your hair. Coconut helps your hair grow thicker, longer, and faster. The vitamins and essential fatty acids naturally found in coconut nourish the scalp and hair follicles.

Jaggery: Jaggery commonly, known as gur in India and Panela in the rest of the world. Regular intake of jaggery in any form with any food will help combat anemia. Jaggery is unrefined sugar; it is the purest form of sugar and is prepared in iron vessels with fruit juices without any addition of synthetic chemicals. It is rich in iron and folate, which help prevent anemia and prevent hair loss, even promote new hair formation.

ABOUT THE AUTHOR

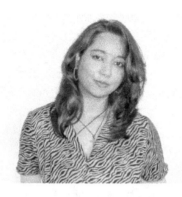

La Fonceur is a dance artist, a health blogger and the author of the book series *Eat So What*. She has a master's degree in Pharmacy, and she is specialized in Pharmaceutical Technology. She has published a review article titled 'Techniques for Producing Biotechnology-Derived Products of Pharmaceutical Use' in Pharmtechmedica Journal. She is a registered state pharmacist. She is a national-level GPAT qualifier of the year 2011 in which she was among the top 1400 nationwide. Being a research scientist, she has worked closely with drugs. Based on her experience, she believes vegetarian foods are the remedy for many diseases; one can prevent most of the diseases with nutritional foods and a healthy lifestyle.

NOTE FROM LA FONCEUR

Thank you for reading this book. I am glad to find someone as health-conscious as much as I am. Being a Lacto Vegetarian, I always look for the healthy vegetarian food options to include in my diet. You can find everything about vegetarian foods in my previous books, **Eat so what! Smart Ways To Stay Healthy** and **Eat so what! The Power of Vegetarianism.** You will learn macronutrients importance, their source, and how plant-based vegetarian foods are the solution to a disease-free healthy life. These books are available in Paperback as well as in Ebook edition in all leading online book stores.

I hope you have found my book useful. I would really appreciate it if you review my book; this will encourage me to write more health books.

La Fonceur

OTHER BOOKS BY LA FONCEUR

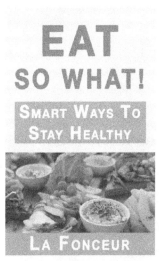
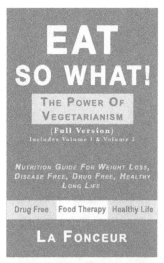
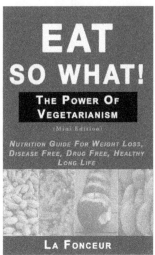
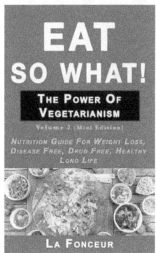

CONNECT WITH LA FONCEUR

Instagram: **@la_fonceur** | **@eatsowhat**

Facebook: **LaFonceur** | **eatsowhat**

Twitter: **@la_fonceur**

Amazon Author Page:

www.amazon.com/La-Fonceur/e/B07PM8SBSG/

Bookbub Author Page: www.bookbub.com/authors/la-fonceur

Sign up to my website to get exclusive offers on my books:

www.lafonceur.com/sign-up

www.eatsowhat.com

CPSIA information can be obtained
at www.ICGtesting.com
Printed in the USA
LVHW091602230321
682224LV00044B/852